Easy Anti Inflammatory Diet Cookbook

Delicious and Tasty Dessert Recipes to Enjoy your Meals

Zac Gibson

1

Citrus cauliflower cake

Prep Time:
5 hours and 30 minutes
Cook Time:
0 minutes
Serve: 10

Ingredients:

For the Crust:

- cup dates, pitted 2½-cups pecan nuts
- Tbsps maple syrup or agave

For the Filling:

- ½-tsp lemon extract
- ½-tsp pure vanilla extract
- ¾-cup maple syrup or agave
- 1½-cups pineapple, crushed
- 1½-cups plain coconut yogurt
- 1-pc lemon, zest, and juice
- 1-tsp pure vanilla extract
- 3-cups cauliflower, riced
- 3-pcs avocados, halved and pitted
- 3-Tbsps maple syrup or agave
- A pinch of cinnamon

Directions:

For the Crust:

1.Coat a baking tray using parchment paper. Set the outer ring of a 9- inch springform pan onto the baking tray.

2.Pulse the pecans in a food processor to a thoroughly ground texture. Put in the remaining crust ingredients, and pulse further until the mixture holds together.

3.Move and press the mixture to a uniform layer in the baking tray.

For the Filling:

1.Wipe the container of your food processor, and put in in the avocado, cauliflower, pineapple, syrup, and lemon zest and juice. Process the mixture to a smooth consistency.

2.Put in the cinnamon and the lemon and vanilla extracts. Pulse until meticulously blended. Pour the mixture over the crust. Put the tray in your freezer overnight, or for around five hours.

3.Take the cake out from your freezer, and allow it to sit at room temperature for about twenty minutes. Take away the outer ring.

For the Topping:

1.Mix in all the topping ingredients in a mixing container. Pour the mixture over the cake and spread uniformly.

Nutrition: ‖ Calories: 667 ‖ Fat: 22.2g ‖ Protein: 33.3g ‖ Sodium: 237mg ‖ Total Carbohydrates: 88.1g ‖ Fiber: 4.8g ‖ Net Carbohydrates: 83.3g

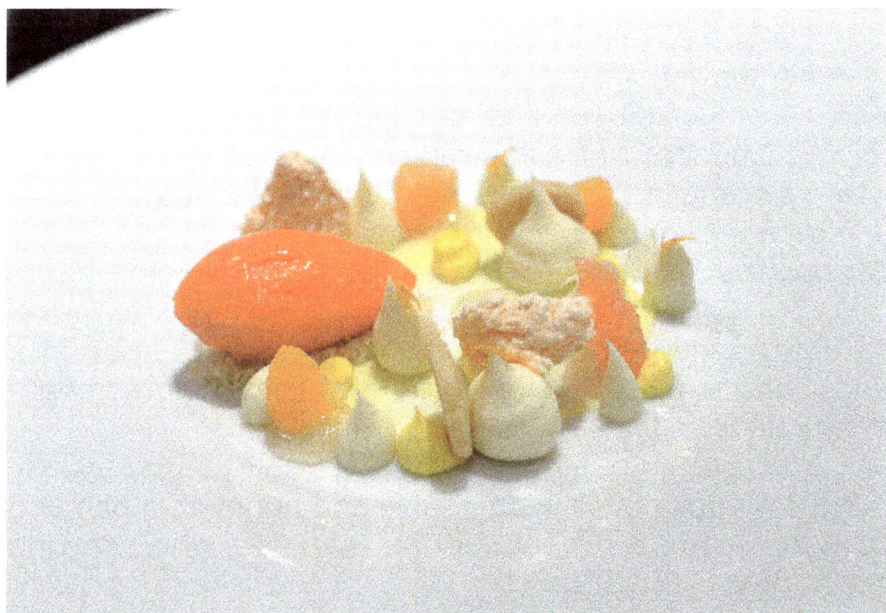

Citrus strawberry granita

Prep Time:
15 minutes
Cook Time:
0 minutes
Serve: 4

Ingredients:

- ¼ cup of raw honey
- ¼ lemon
- 1 grapefruit (peeled, seeded, and sectioned)
- 12 ounces of fresh strawberries, hulled
- 2 oranges (peeled, seeded and sectioned)

Directions:

1.Put strawberries, grapefruit, oranges, and lemon in a juicer and extract juice according to the manufacturer's instructions.

2.Put 1½ cups of the veggie juice and honey to a pan and cook on moderate heat for five minutes while stirring constantly.

3.Remove it from heat and put in it to the rest of the juice.

4.Set aside for roughly thirty minutes.

5.Move the juice mixture into an 8x8-inch glass baking dish.

6.Freeze for 4 hours while scraping after every thirty minutes.

Nutrition: ‖ Calories: 145 ‖ Fat: 0.4g ‖ Carbohydrates: 37.5g ‖ Sugar: 32.4g ‖ Protein: 1.7g ‖ Sodium: 2mg

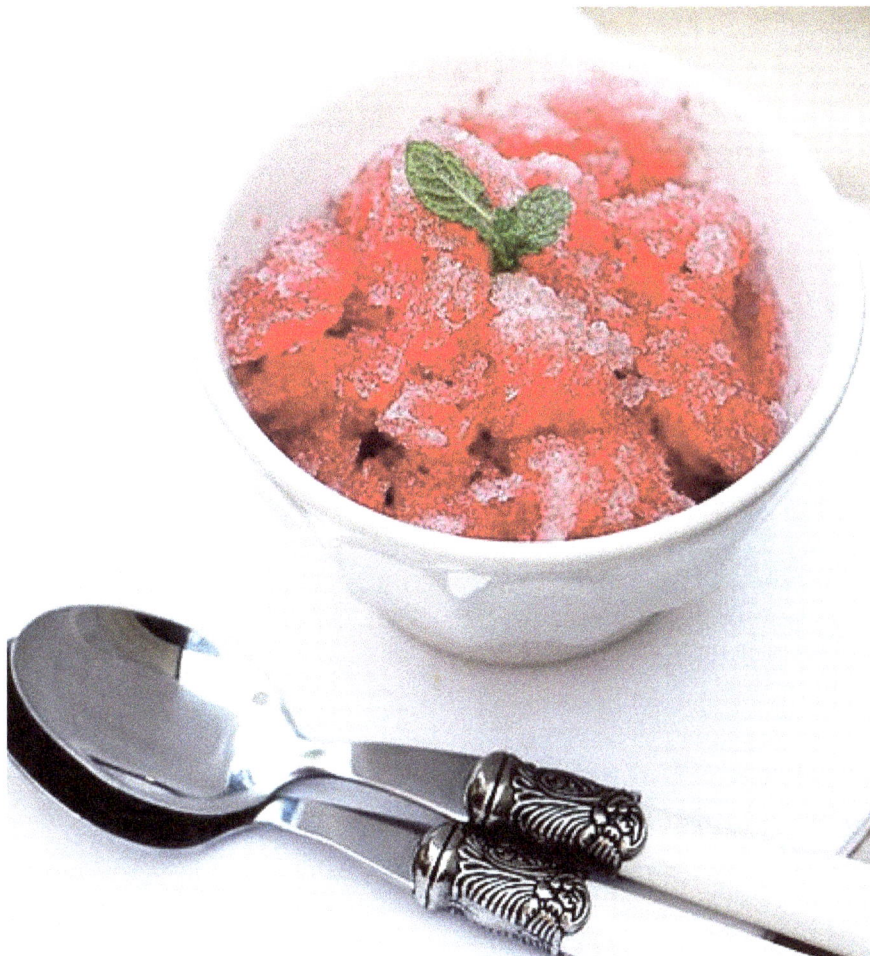

Coconut and chocolate cream

Prep Time:
2 hours
Cook Time:
0 minutes
Serve: 4

Ingredients:

- ½ teaspoon cinnamon powder
- 1cup dark chocolate, chopped and melted
- 1 teaspoon vanilla extract
- 2cups coconut milk
- 2 tablespoons ginger, grated
- 2 tablespoons honey

Directions:

1.Throw all the ingredients into a blender and blend. Split into bowls and store in the refrigerator for about two hours before you serve.

Nutrition: ‖ Calories: 200 ‖ Fat: 3 ‖ Fiber:5 ‖ Carbohydrates: 12 ‖ Protein: 7

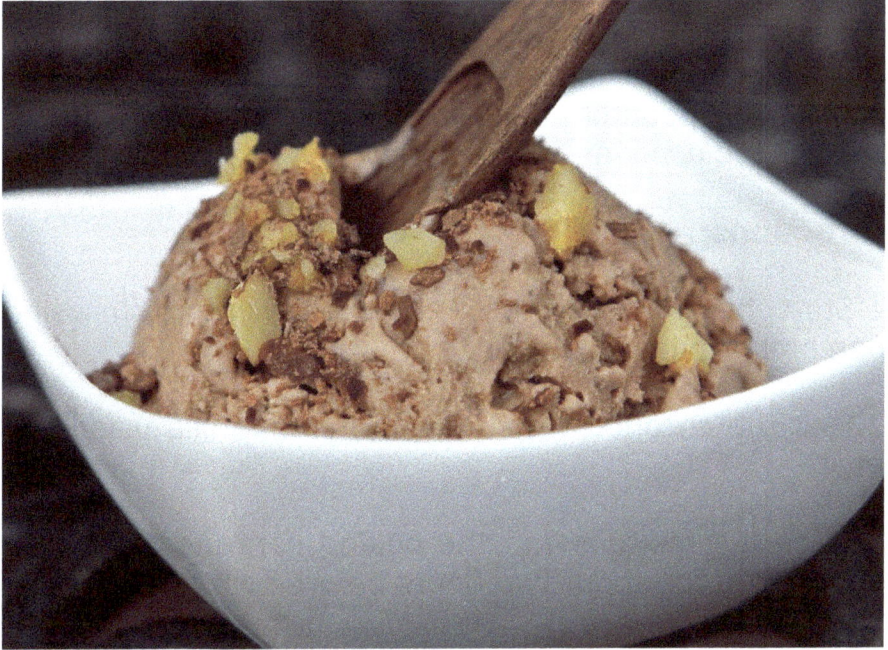

Coconut butter fudge

Prep Time:
10 minutes
Cook Time:
0 minutes
Serve: 6

Ingredients:

- ¼ teaspoon of salt
- 1 cup of coconut butter
- 1 teaspoon of pure vanilla extract
- 2 tablespoons of raw honey

Directions:

1.Start by lining an 8 x 8 inch baking dish using parchment paper.

2.Melt the coconut butter, honey, and vanilla using low heat.

3.Place the mixture into the baking pan and place it in your fridge for about two hours before serving.

Nutrition: ‖ Total Carbohydrates: 6g ‖ Fiber: 0g ‖ Net Carbohydrates: ‖ Protein: 0g ‖ Total Fat: 36g ‖ Calories: 334

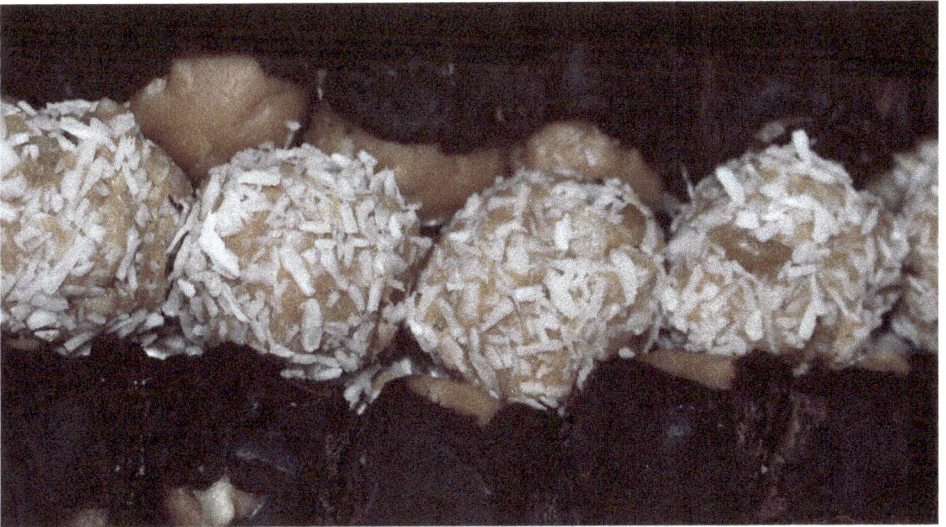

Coconut muffins

Prep Time:
5 minutes
Cook Time:
25 minutes
Serve: 8

Ingredients:

- ¼ cup of cocoa powder
- ¼ teaspoon vanilla extract
- ½ cup ghee, melted
- 1 cup coconut, unsweetened and shredded
- 1 teaspoon baking powder
- 3 tablespoons swerve eggs, whisked

Directions:

1.In a container, mix the ghee with the swerve, coconut, and the other ingredients, stir thoroughly and split it into a lined muffin pan.

2.Bake at 370 degrees F for about twenty-five minutes, cool down before you serve.

Nutrition: ‖ Calories: 324 ‖ Fat: 31g ‖ Carbohydrates: 8.3g ‖ Protein: 4g ‖ Sugar: 11g

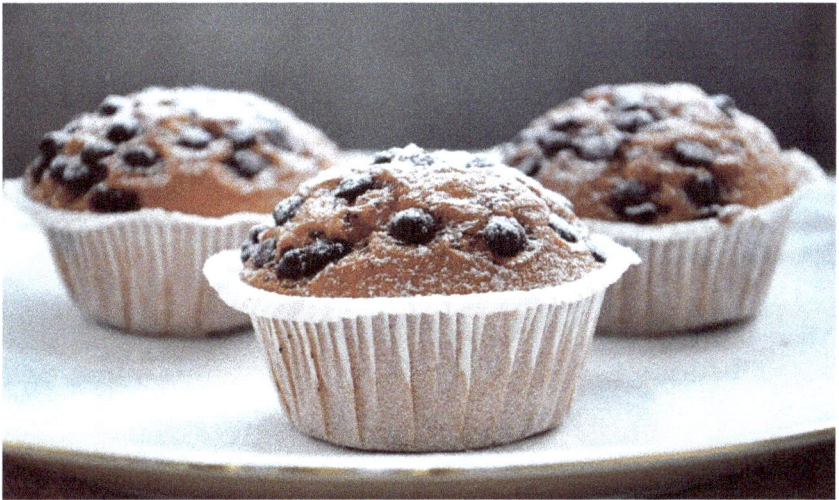

Coffee Cream

Prep Time:
10 minutes
Cook Time:
15 minutes
Serve: 4

Ingredients:

- ¼ cup brewed coffee
- 1 teaspoon vanilla extract
- 2 cups heavy cream
- 2 eggs
- 2 tablespoons ghee, melted
- 2 tablespoons swerve

Directions:

1.In a container, mix the coffee with the cream and the other ingredients, whisk well and split it into 4 ramekins and whisk well.

2.Introduce the ramekins in your oven at 350 degrees F and bake for fifteen minutes.

Nutrition: Calories 300 ‖ Fat: 11g ‖ Carbohydrates: 3g ‖ Protein: 4g ‖ Sugar: 12g

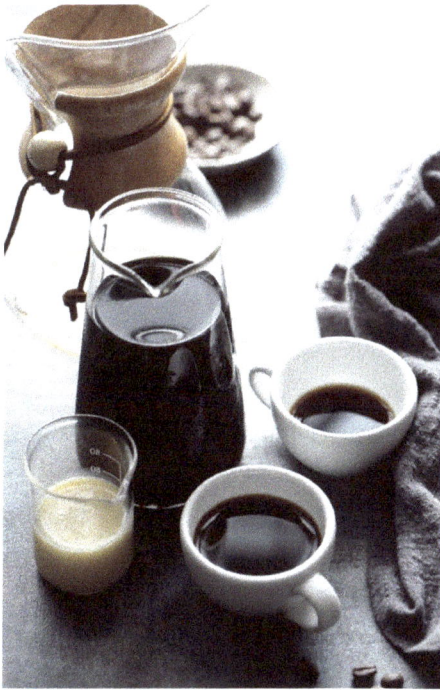
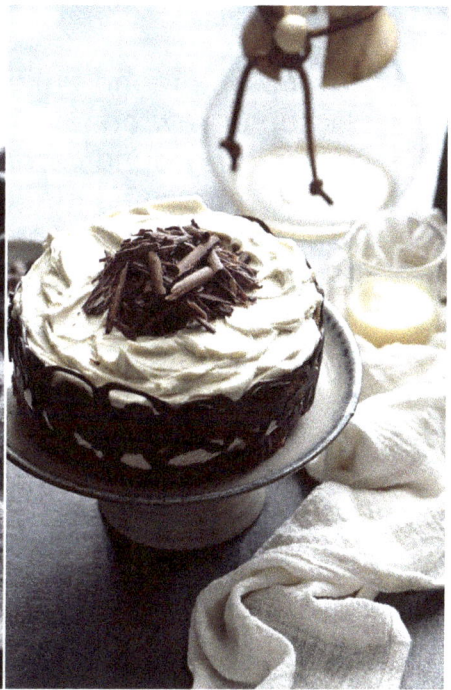

Comforting Baked Rice Pudding

Prep Time:
10 minutes
Cook Time:
20 minutes
Serve: 8

Ingredients:

- ¼ cup of almond flakes
- ¼ cup of raw honey
- ½ tsp. of ground cardamom
- ½ tsp. of ground ginger
- 1 peeled and cut banana
- 1 tsp. fresh lemon zest, finely grated
- 1 tsp. of ground cinnamon
- 2 big organic eggs
- 2 cups of cooked brown rice
- 2 cups of unsweetened almond milk

Directions:

1. Set the oven to 390 F, then grease a baking dish.

2. Spread cooked rice at the bottom of the readied baking dish uniformly.

3. In a big container, put together the coconut milk, eggs, honey, lemon zest, spices, and beat until well blended.

4. Put the egg mixture over the rice uniformly.

5. Position banana slices over egg mixture uniformly and drizzle with almonds.

6. Bake for approximately twenty minutes.

Nutrition: ‖ Calories: 264 ‖ Fat: 4.9g ‖ Carbohydrates: 50g ‖ Protein: 6.2g ‖ Fiber: 2.9g

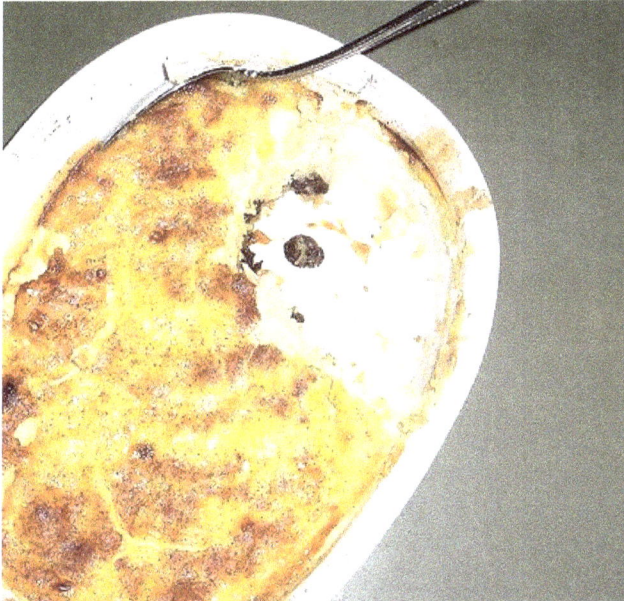

Cookie Dough Bites

Prep Time:
10 minutes
Cook Time:
5 minutes
Serve: 2

Ingredients:

- ¼ cup Almond Flour
- ¼ cup Chocolate Chips, dairy-free & sugar-free
- ½ cup Almond Butter or any nut butter
- ½ tsp. Salt
- 1 ½ cups Chickpeas, cooked
- 1 tsp. Vanilla Extract
- 2 tbsp. Maple Syrup

Directions:

1. First, place all the ingredients excluding the chocolate chips in a high-speed blender for about three minutes or until you get a thick, smooth mixture.

2. After this, move the mixture to a moderate-sized container.

3. Next, fold in the chocolate chips into the batter.

4. Check for sweetness and put in more maple syrup if required.

Nutrition: ‖ Calories: 373 Kcal ‖ Protein: 12.6g ‖ Carbohydrates: 59.1g ‖ Fat:10g

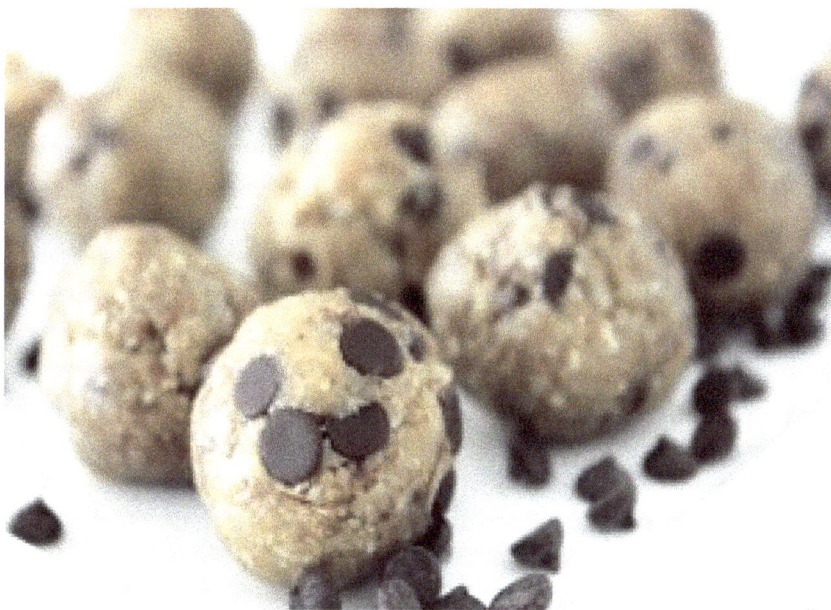

Creamy & Chilly Blueberry Bites

Prep Time:
2 hours and 5 minutes
Cook Time:
0 minutes
Serve: 2

Ingredients:

- 1-pint blueberries 2-tsp lemon juice
- 8-oz. vanilla yogurt

Directions:

1.Coat the blueberries with the lemon juice and yogurt in a mixing container. Toss cautiously without squishing the berries.

2.Scoop out each of the coated berries and arrange them on a baking sheet coated with parchment paper. Place the sheet in your freezer for a couple of hours before you serve.

Nutrition: ‖ Calories: 394 ‖ Fat: 13.1g ‖ Protein: 19.7g ‖ Sodium: 164mg ‖ Total Carbohydrates: 58.9g ‖ Fiber: 9.7g ‖ Net Carbohydrates: 49.2g

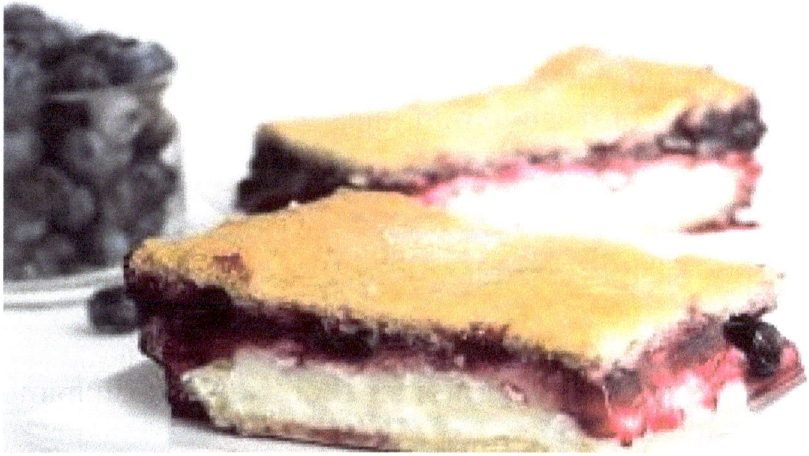

Creamy Frozen Yogurt

Prep Time:
10 minutes + 2-3 hours freezing
Serve: Servings 3

Ingredients:

- ½ cup of coconut yogurt
- ½ cup of unsweetened almond milk
- 1 tbsp. of raw honey
- 1 tsp. of fresh mint leaves
- 1 tsp. of organic vanilla extract
- 2 peeled, pitted and chopped medium avocados
- 2 tbsp. of fresh lemon juice

Directions:

1. Throw all the ingredients into a blender apart from mint leaves and pulse till creamy and smooth.

2. Put into an airtight container then freeze for minimum 2-three hours.

3. Take off from the freezer and keep aside for about fifteen minutes.

4. With a spoon stir thoroughly.

5. Top with fresh mint leaves before you serve.

Nutrition: ‖ Calories: 105 ‖ Fat: 1.3g ‖ Carbohydrates: 20.3g ‖ Protein: 2.8 g ‖ Fiber: 1.4g

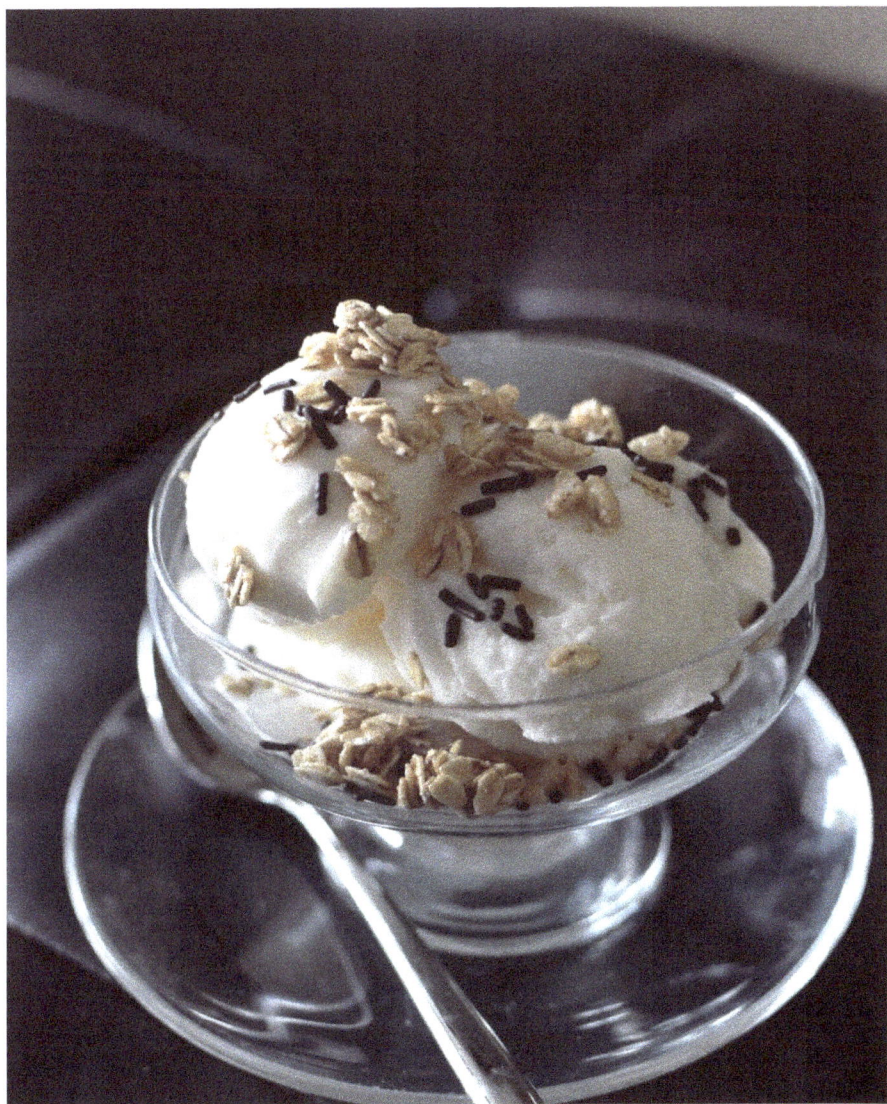

Dark Chocolate Granola Bars

Prep Time:
10 minutes
Cook Time:
25 minutes
Serve: 12

Ingredients:

- ¼ cup dark cocoa powder
- ¼ cup of flaxseed
- ½ cup dark chocolate chips
- 1 cup of walnuts
- 1 cup tart cherries, dried
- 1 teaspoon of salt
- 1 teaspoon of vanilla
- 2 cups buckwheat
- 2 eggs
- 2/3 cup honey

Directions:

1.Preheat the oven to 350 degrees F.

2.Line with cooking spray your baking pan.

3.Pulse together the walnuts, wheat, tart cherries, salt, and flaxseed in a food processor. Everything must be chopped fine.

4.Mix the honey, eggs, vanilla, and cocoa powder in a container.

5.Put in the wheat mix to your container. Stir to blend well.

6.Include the chocolate chips. Stir once more.

7.Now pour this mixture into a baking dish.

8.Drizzle some chocolate chips and tart cherries.

9.Bake for about twenty-five minutes. Allow to cool before you serve.

Nutrition: Calories 364 ‖ Carbohydrates: 37g ‖ Cholesterol: 60mg ‖ Fat: 20g ‖ Protein: 6g ‖ Sugar: 22g ‖ Fiber: 4g ‖ Sodium: 214mg

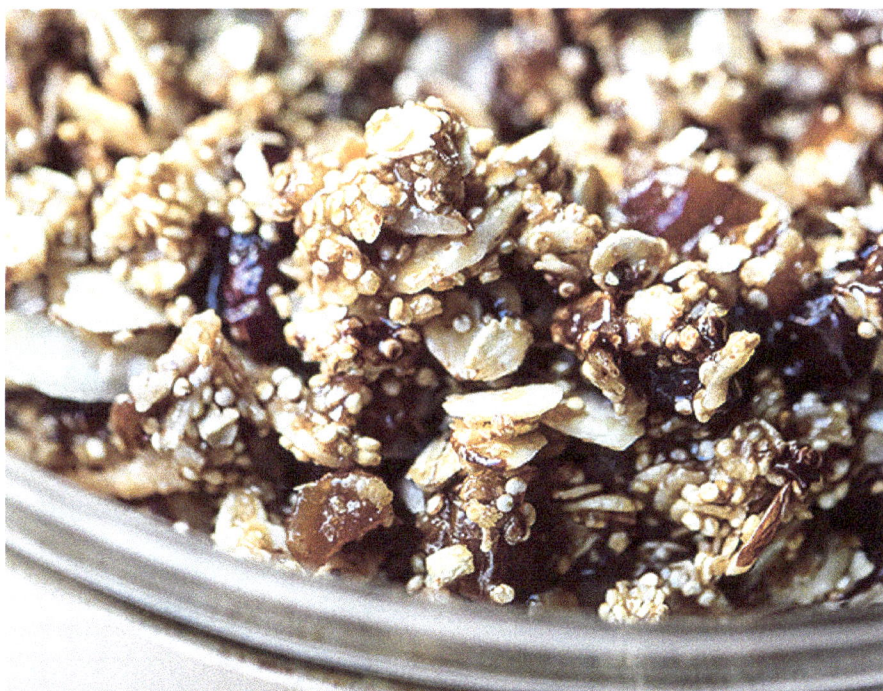

Date Dough & Walnut Wafer

Prep Time:
15 minutes
Cook Time:
18 minutes
Serve: 8

Ingredients:

- ¼-cup coconut oil
- ¼-tsp sea salt
- ½-cup coconut, unsweetened
- ½-cup walnuts
- ½-tsp baking soda
- ½-tsp sea salt
- 1½-cup oats (divided)
- 18-pcs Medjool dates, pitted
- 1-pc egg
- 1-tsp lemon juice
- 2-Tbsps ground flaxseed
- 6-pcs Medjool dates, pitted and cut into four equivalent portions

Directions:

1.Preheat the oven to 325ºF. Coat a baking pan using parchment paper.

2.Pulse a cup of oats in a food processor until making a flour consistency.

3.Put in in the dates, coconut, baking soda, and sea salt. Pulse again until the dates completely break up.

4.Put in the remaining oats and walnuts, and pulse until the nuts break, but still a bit lumpy. Put in the flaxseed, egg, and oil. Pulse the mixture further until meticulously blended.

5.Set aside ½-cup of the date mixture to use as a topping later. Push down the rest of the mix to a uniform layer in the pan.

6.Wash your food processor, and put in all the date layer ingredients. Pulse the mixture until the dates completely break up and take on a light caramel color.

7.With wet hands, press the mixture down, smoothing it on the date mixture. Crumble and drizzle the reserved date mixture over the top.

8.Place the pan in your oven. Bake for eighteen minutes. Allow the wafer to cool to room temperature before cutting into 16 pieces.

Nutrition: ‖ Calories: 203 ‖ Fat: 6.7g ‖ Protein: 10.1g ‖ Sodium: 76mg ‖ Total Carbohydrates: 28.3g ‖ Fiber: 3g ‖ Net Carbohydrates: 25.3g

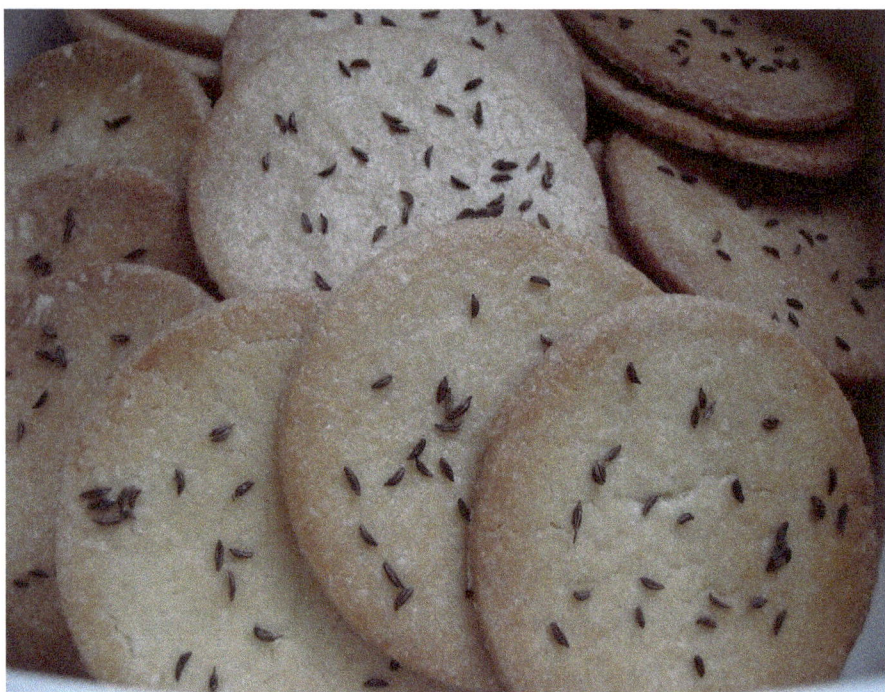

Easy Peach Cobbler

Prep Time:
5 minutes
Cook Time:
20 minutes
Serve: 6

Ingredients:

- ¼ brown rice flour
- ¼ cup coconut palm sugar, divided
- ¼ cup extra virgin olive oil
- ¼ cup ground flaxseeds
- ½ cup gluten-free oats
- ½ teaspoon cinnamon
- ¾ cup chopped pecans
- 5 organic peaches, pitted and chopped

Directions:

1.Preheat your oven to 3500F.

2.Grease the bottom of 6 ramekins.

3.In a container, combine the peaches, ½ of the coconut sugar, cinnamon, and pecans.

4.Distribute the peach mixture into the ramekins.

5.In the same container, combine the oats, flaxseed, rice flour, and oil. Put in in the rest of the coconut sugar. Mix until a crumbly texture is formed.

6.Top the mixture over the peaches.

7.Put for about twenty minutes.

Nutrition: Calories 26 ‖ Fat: 11g ‖ Carbohydrates: 28g ‖ Protein: 10g ‖ Sugar: 12g ‖ Fiber: 6g

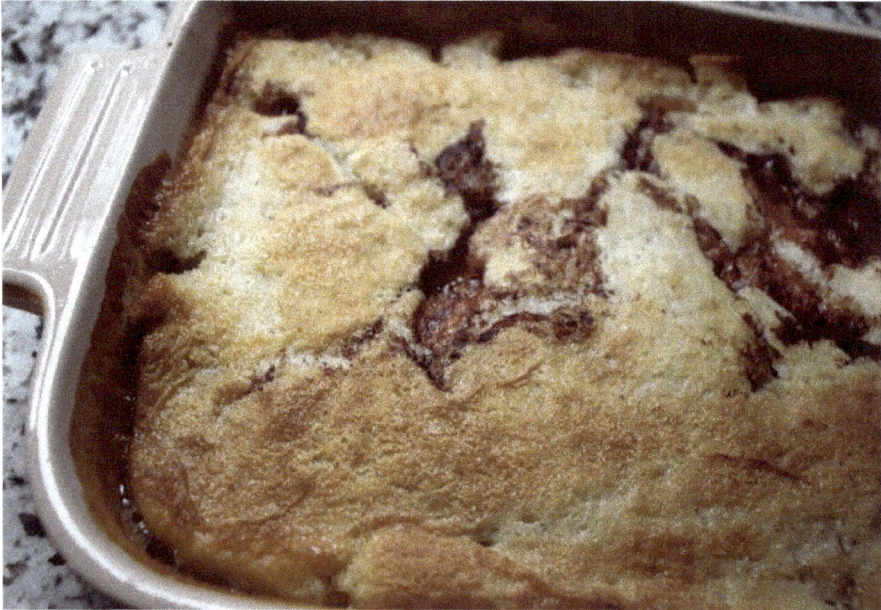

Fall-Time Custard

Prep Time:
15 minutes
Cook Time:
60 minutes
Serve: 6

Ingredients:

- ¼ tsp. of ground ginger
- 1 cup of canned pumpkin
- 1 cup of coconut milk
- 1 tsp. of ground cinnamon
- 1 tsp. of organic vanilla extract
- 2 organic eggs
- 2pinches of freshly grated nutmeg 8-10 drops of liquid stevia
- Pinch of salt

Directions:

1.Preheat your oven to 350 degrees F.

2.In a big container, put together pumpkin and spices then mix.

3.In another container, put in the eggs and beat thoroughly.

4.Put in the rest of the ingredients then whisk till well blended.

5.Put in egg mixture into pumpkin mixture and mix till well blended.

6.Move the mixture toto 6 ramekins.

7.Position the ramekins in a baking dish,

8.Put in sufficient water in the baking dish about two-inch high around the ramekins.

9.Bake for approximately 1 hour or till a toothpick inserted in the middle comes out clean.

Nutrition: ‖ Calories: 131 ‖ Fat: 11.1g ‖ Carbohydrates: 6.1g ‖ Protein: 3.3g ‖ Fiber: 2.3g

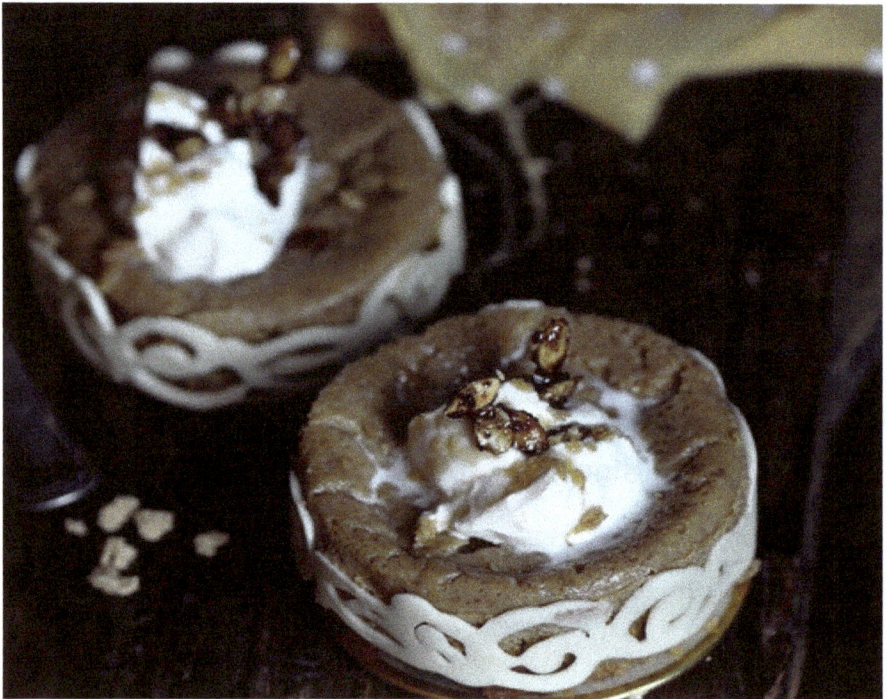

Fennel And Almond Bites

Prep Time:
10 minutes
 + 3 hours freezing time
Cook Time:
25 minutes
Serve: 10

Ingredients:

- ¼ cup almond milk
- ¼ cup of cocoa powder
- ½ cup almond oil
- 1 teaspoon fennel seeds
- 1 teaspoon vanilla extract
- A pinch of sunflower seeds

Directions:

1.Take a container and mix the almond oil and almond milk

2.Beat until the desired smoothness is achieved and shiny by using an electric beater. Stir in the remaining ingredients

3.Take a piping bag and pour into a parchment paper-lined baking sheet

4.Freeze for around three hours and stored in your refrigerator

Nutrition: ‖ Total Carbohydrates: 1g ‖ Fiber: 1g ‖ Protein: 1g ‖ Fat: 20g

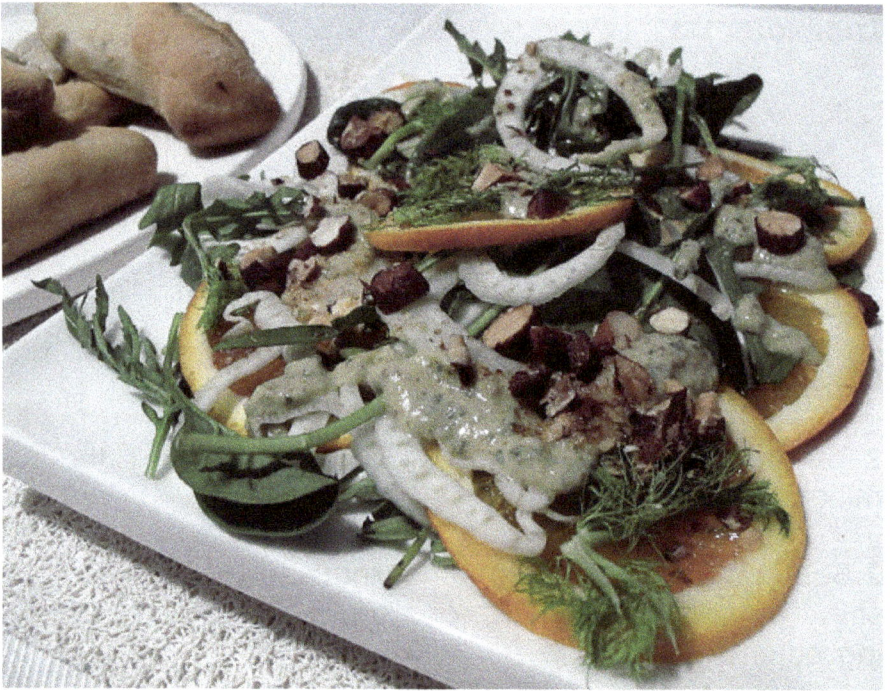

Flourless Sweet Potato Brownies

Prep Time:
10 minutes
 Cook Time:
30 minutes
Serve: 9

Ingredients:

- ¼ cup Unsweetened Cocoa powder
- ½ cup Almond butter
- ½ cup Cooked sweet potato
- ½ tsp. Baking soda
- 1 big Whole egg
- 2 tsp. Vanilla extract
- 3 tbsp. Dairy-free chocolate chips, optional.
- 6 tbsp. Honey

Directions:

1. Prep the oven by preheating to 350ºF.

2. Coat a baking pan using parchment paper leaving a few extra inches on the sides to make it easier to discard or remove

3. Blend all the ingredients, excluding the chocolate chips until you get a super smooth and tender batter.

4. Move the creamy batter to your readied baking pan and use a spatula to spread it around, so it looks almost even.

5. Slide it in your oven, then bake for thirty minutes or until a knife inserted into the pan comes out clean.

6. Remove from the oven and leave to cool in the pan for fifteen minutes before putting it up on a wire rack.

7. If you decide to use the chocolate chip topping, put the chips in a microwave-safe dish and heat until it completely melts.

8.Remove from the microwave and sprinkle over the brownies.

Nutrition: ‖ Calories: 171 kcal ‖ Protein: 5.17 g ‖ Fat: 9.28 g ‖ Carbohydrates: 20.01 g

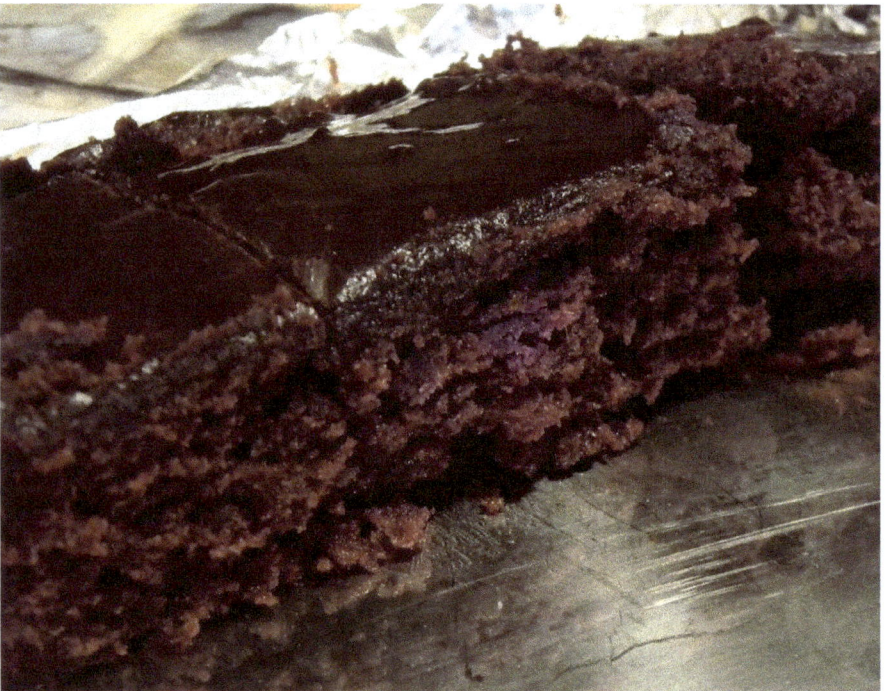

Fried Pineapple Slice

Prep Time:
10 minutes
Cook Time:
8 minutes
Serve: 8

Ingredients:

- ¼ cup of coconut oil
- ¼ cup of coconut palm sugar
- ¼ teaspoon of ground cinnamon
- 1 fresh pineapple (peeled and slice into big slices)

Directions:

1. Warm a huge cast-iron frying pan on moderate heat.

2. Put in oil and sugar and cook until the coconut oil has melted while stirring constantly.

3. Put in the pineapple slices into two batches and cook for roughly 1- 2 minutes.

4. Flip the medial side and cook for approximately one minute. Carry on cooking for one more minute.

5. Repeat the steps with the rest of the slices.

6. Drizzle with cinnamon before you serve.

Nutrition: ‖ Calories: 138 ‖ Fat: 7g ‖ Carbohydrates: 20.9g ‖ Sugar: 15.7g ‖ Protein: 0.6g ‖ Sodium: 15mg

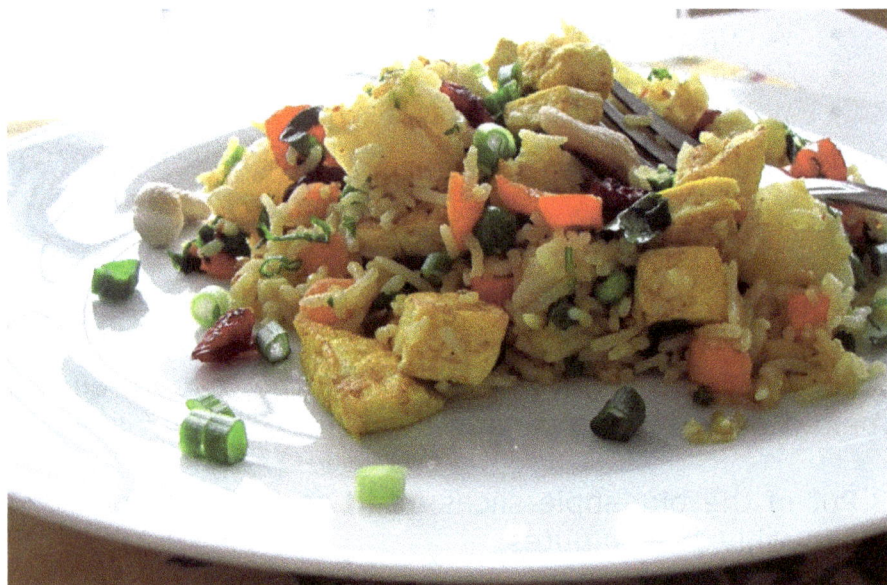

Fruit Cobbler

Prep Time:
10 minutes
Cook Time:
 20 minutes
Serve:8

Ingredients:

- ¼ Cup Coconut Oil, Melted
- ¼ Cup Coconut Sugar
- ½ Teaspoon Vanilla Extract, Pure
- ¾ Cup Almond Flour
- ¾ Cup Rolled Oats
- 1 Teaspoon Coconut Oil
- 1 Teaspoon Ground Cinnamon
- 2 Cups Nectarines, Fresh & Sliced
- 2 Cups Peaches, Fresh & Sliced
- 2 Tablespoons Lemon Juice, Fresh Dash Salt
- Filter Water for Mixing

Directions:

1.Begin by heating the oven to 425.

2.Get out a cast-iron frying pan, coating it with a teaspoon of coconut oil.

3.Mix your lemon juice, peaches, and nectarines in the frying pan.

4.Prepare your food processor, mixing your almond flour, oats, coconut sugar, and remaining coconut oil.

5.Put in in your cinnamon, vanilla, and salt, pulsing until the oat mixture looks like a dry dough.

6.If you need more moisture, put in filtered water a tablespoon at a time, and then break the dough into chunks, spreading it across the fruit.

7.Bake for 20 minutes before you serve warm.

Nutrition: ‖ Protein: 4 Grams ‖ Fat: 12 Grams ‖ Carbohydrates: fifteen Grams

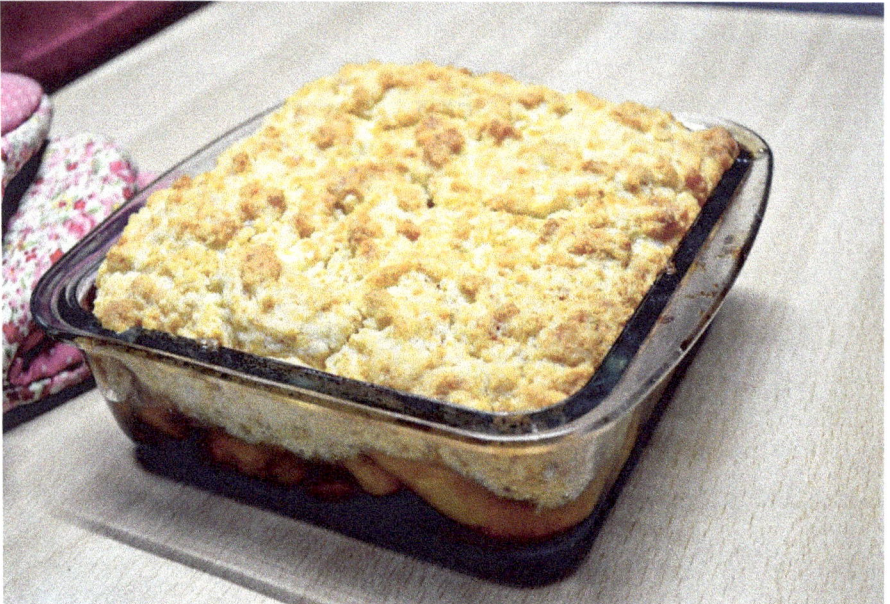

Fruit Salad

Prep Time:
10 minutes
Cook Time:
20 minutes
Serve: 2-3

Ingredients:

- ½ of 1 Watermelon, chopped into little pieces
- 1 Pineapple, cut into little pieces
- 1 Pomegranate, small
- 1 Red Papaya, cut into little pieces
- 1 tsp. Ginger, freshly grated
- 4 Strawberries, chopped Dash of Turmeric

Directions:

1. To start with, place all the fruits in a large-sized container.

2. Next, spoon in the turmeric and ginger over the fruits.

3. Toss thoroughly before you serve.

Nutrition: ‖ Calories: 118Kcal ‖ Protein: 1.6g ‖ Carbohydrates: 36.6g ‖ Fat: 0.5g

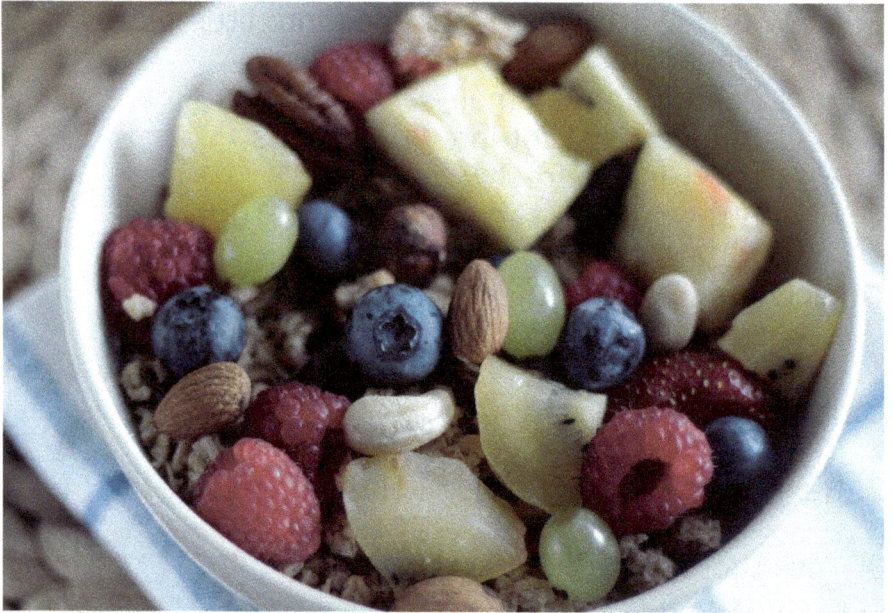

Glazed Banana

Prep Time:
10 minutes
Cook Time:
5 minutes
Serve: 2

Ingredients:

- 1 peeled and cut under-ripened banana
- 1 tbsp. of filtered water
- 1 tbsp. of olive oil
- 1 tbsp. of raw honey
- 1/8 tsp. of ground cinnamon

Directions:

1.In a nonstick frying pan, warm oil on moderate heat.

2.Put in banana slices and cook for approximately 1-2 minutes per side.

3.In the meantime, in a small container, put in water and honey and beat thoroughly.

4.Move the banana slices on a serving plate.

5.Instantly, pour honey mixture over banana slices.

6.Keep aside to cool to room temperature. Serve with the drizzling of cinnamon.

Nutrition: ‖ Calories: 145 ‖ Fat: 7.2g ‖ Carbohydrates: 22.2g ‖ Protein: 0.7g ‖ Fiber: 1.6g

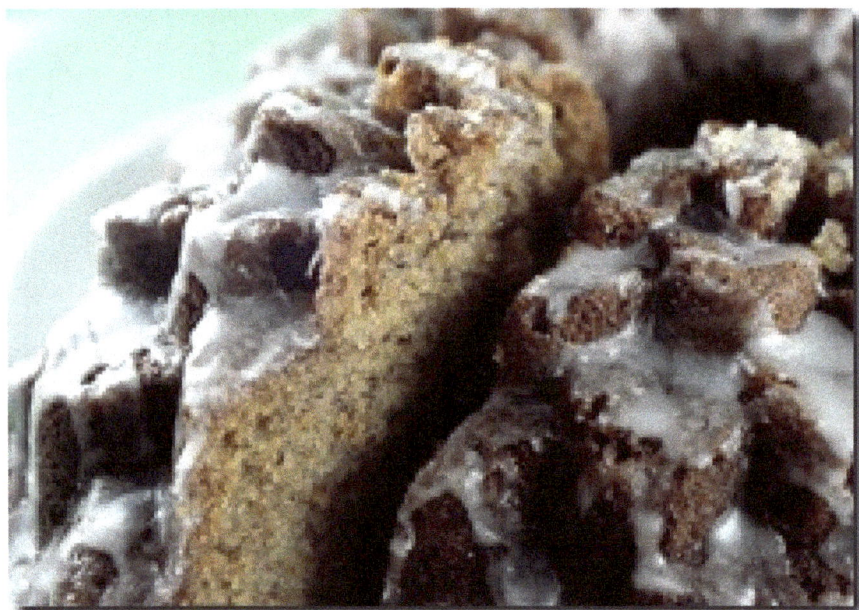

Glorious Blueberry Crumble

Prep Time:
10 minutes
Cook Time:
30 minutes
Serve: 6

Ingredients:

- ½ cup of softened coconut oil
- ½ tsp. of ground cinnamon
- 1 cup of almond meal
- 1 cup of toasted and finely crushed almonds
- 2 tbsp. of coconut sugar
- 4 cups of fresh blueberries

Directions:

1.Set the oven to 350F then lightly, grease a pie dish.

2.In a huge container, combine all ingredients apart from blueberries.

3.Split half of the almond mixture at the bottom of the prepared pie dish.

4.Put blueberries over almond mixture uniformly.

5.Top with the rest of the almond mixture uniformly.

6.Bake for minimum 30 minutes or till the top becomes golden brown.

Nutrition: ‖ Calories: 411 ‖ Fat: 34.3g ‖ Carbohydrates: 24.9g ‖ Protein: 7.4g ‖ Fiber: 6.4g

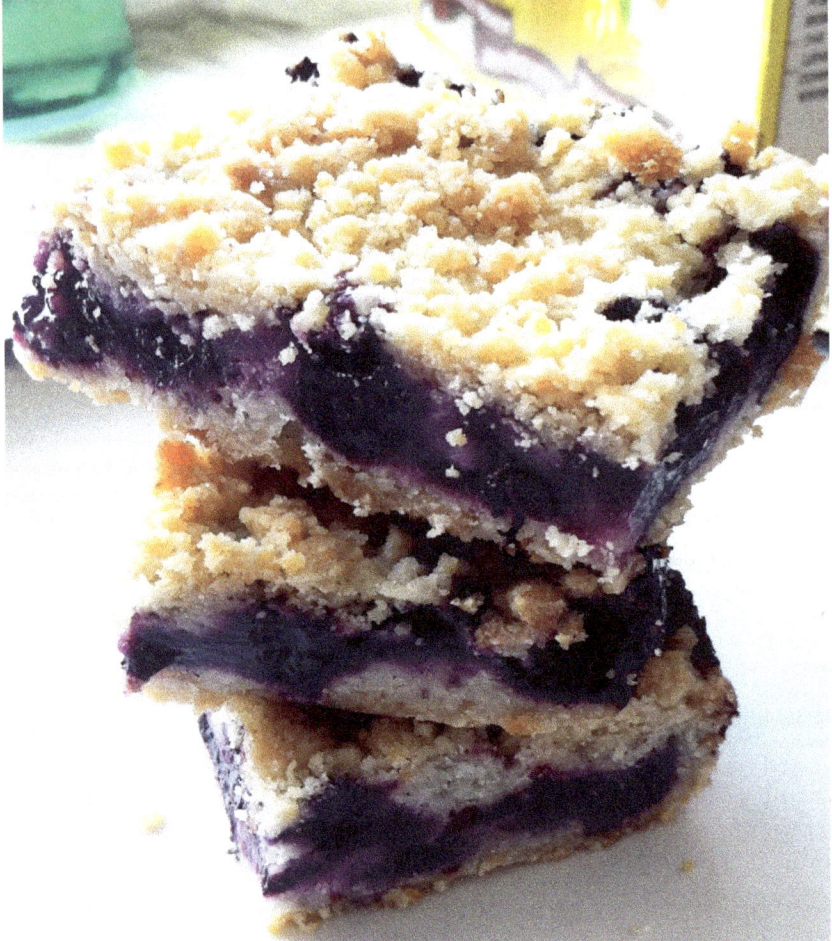

Green Tea Pudding

Prep Time:
20 minutes
Cook Time:
10 minutes
Serve: 3

Ingredients:

- 1 Tsp. Matcha Green Tea Powder
- 1/4 Cup Brown Sugar
- 1/4 Cup Corn Starch
- 1/8-Tbsp. Cinnamon Powder 100g Butter
- 2 Cup Heavy Milk
- 3 Eggs
- Salt

Directions:

1.In a big pot, mix brown sugar, milk, cornstarch, and matcha powder.

2.In moderate heat, keep whisking until combined.

3.Combine the hot batter with whisked eggs slowly.

4.Cook for three to five minutes.

5.Strain the mixture and put in butter.

6.Place the mixture in a container and place in your fridge for a few hours before serving.

Nutrition: ‖ Calories: 359 kcal ‖ Carbohydrates: 60 g ‖ Fat: 3.0 g ‖ Protein: 18.4 g

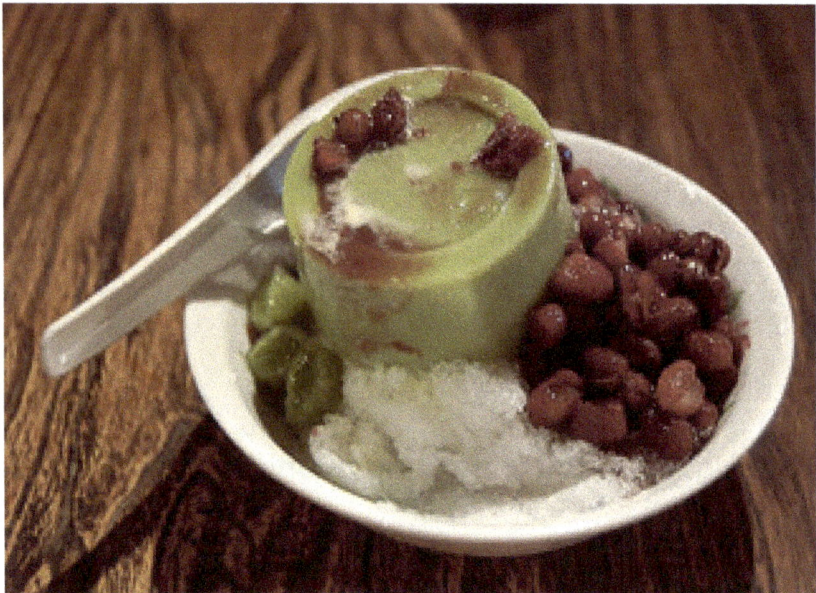

Grilled Peaches

Prep Time:
10 minutes
Cook Time:
10 minutes
Serve: 6

Ingredients:

- ¼ cup of walnuts, chopped
- ½ cup of coconut cream
- 1 teaspoon of organic vanilla extract
- 3 medium peaches (halved and pitted)
- Ground cinnamon

Directions:

1.Preheat the grill on moderate to low heat. Grease the grill grate.

2.Position the peach slices on the grill with the cut-side down.

3.Grill each side for three to five minutes or until the desired doneness is attained.

4.In the meantime, mix coconut cream with vanilla extract in a container. Beat until the desired smoothness is achieved.

5.Ladle the whipped cream over each peach half.

6.Top with walnuts and drizzle with cinnamon.

Nutrition: ‖ Calories: 110 ‖ Fat: 8g ‖ Carbohydrates: 8.8g ‖ Sugar: 7.8g ‖ Protein: 2.4g ‖ Sodium: 3mg

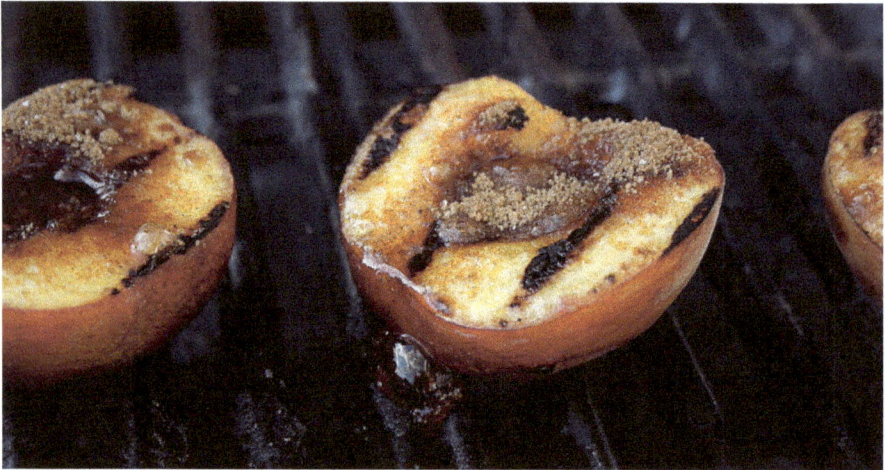

Hot Chocolate

Prep Time:
5 minutes
Cook Time:
5 minutes
Serve: 2

Ingredients:

- ¼ tsp. Turmeric
- ½ tsp. Cinnamon
- 1tbsp. Coconut Oil
- 1 tbsp. Honey, raw
- 2 cups Almond Milk
- 2tbsp. Cocoa Powder, unsweetened

Directions:

1.To start with, bring the almond milk to its boiling point in a deep deep cooking pan on moderate heat.

2.Now, bring this mixture to a simmer and then mix in the cocoa powder to it.

3.Next, spoon in the turmeric powder and cinnamon to it. Mix thoroughly/

4.Next, put in honey to it and once blended well, put in the coconut oil

5.Give the drink a good stir until everything comes together.

Nutrition: ‖ Calories: 150 Kcal ‖ Protein: 2.1g ‖ Carbohydrates: 15.2g ‖ Fat: 11.1gm

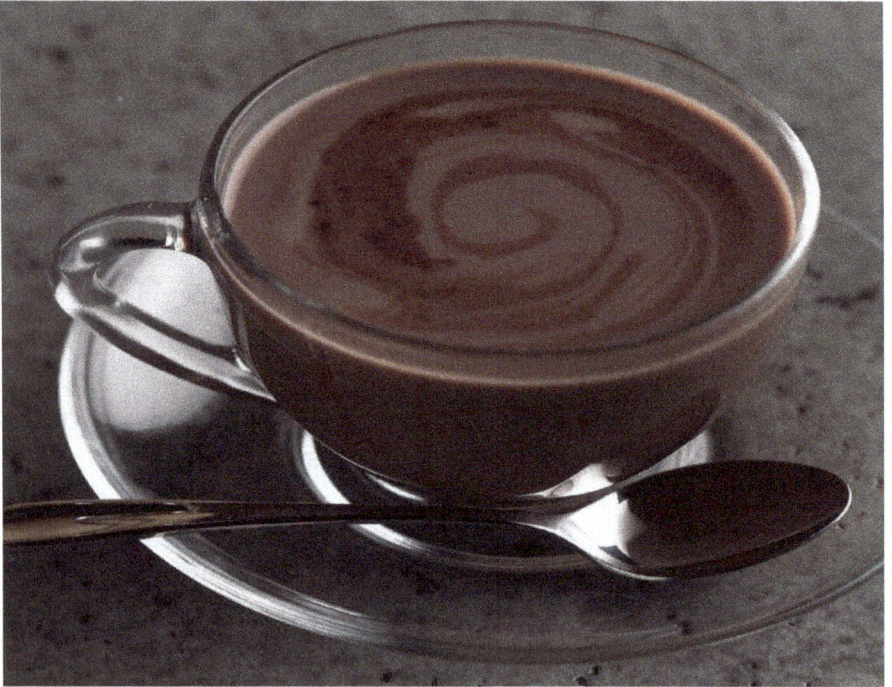

Lemon Sorbet

Prep Time:
10 minutes
Cook Time:
0 minutes
Serve: 2

Ingredients:

- ½ cup of raw honey
- ½ cups of fresh lemon juice
- 2 cups of filtered water
- 2 tablespoons of fresh lemon zest, grated

Directions:

1.Put into your freezer the ice-cream maker tub for a day before making the sorbet.

2.Combine all ingredients in a pan, excluding the freshly squeezed lemon juice and cook on moderate heat.

3.Simmer for minimum 1 minute, up to the sugar dissolves while stirring constantly.

4.Take away the mixture from the heat and put in lemon juice.

5.Move the combination to an airtight container and place in your fridge for around 2hours.

6.Put it into an ice-cream maker and process according to the manufacturer's instructions.

7.Put in one tablespoon of oil when the motor is running.

8.Return the ice-cream into the airtight container and freeze for roughly 2 hours.

Nutrition: ‖ Calories: 305 ‖ Fat: 1.5g ‖ Carbohydrates: 74.9g ‖ Sugar: 73.8g ‖ Protein: 1.9g ‖ Sodium: 40mg

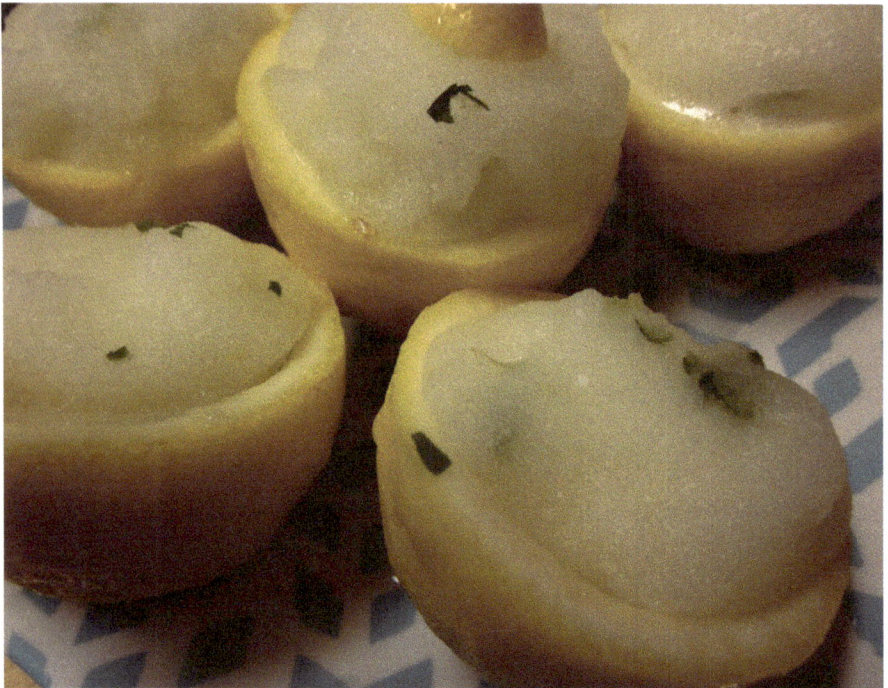

Lemon Vegan Cake

Prep Time:
10 minutes
Cook Time:
10 minutes
Serve: 3

Ingredients:

- ½ lemon extract
- 1 cup of pitted dates
- 1 lemon juice and zest
- 1½ cup agave
- 1½ cups of dairy-free yogurt
- 1½ cups pineapple, crushed
- 1½ teaspoon vanilla extract
- 2½ cups pecans
- 3 avocados, halved & pitted
- 3 cups of cauliflower rice, prepared
- A pinch of cinnamon

Directions:

1. Coat your baking sheet using parchment paper.

2. Pulse the pecans in a food processor.

3. Put in the agave and dates. Pulse for one minute.

4. Move this mix to the baking sheet. Wipe the container of your processor.

5. Combine the pineapple, agave, avocados, cauliflower, lemon juice, and zest in a food processor. Pulse till smooth

6.Now put in the lemon extract, cinnamon, and vanilla extract. Pulse.

7.Pour this mix into your pan, on the crust.

8.Place in your fridge for around five hours at least.

9.Take out the cake and keep it at room temperature for about twenty minutes.

10.Take out the cake's outer ring.

11.Mix the vanilla extract, agave, and yogurt in a container.

12.Pour on your cake.

Nutrition: Calories 688 ǁ Carbohydrates: 100g ǁ Fat: 28g ǁ Protein: 9g ǁ Sugar: 40g

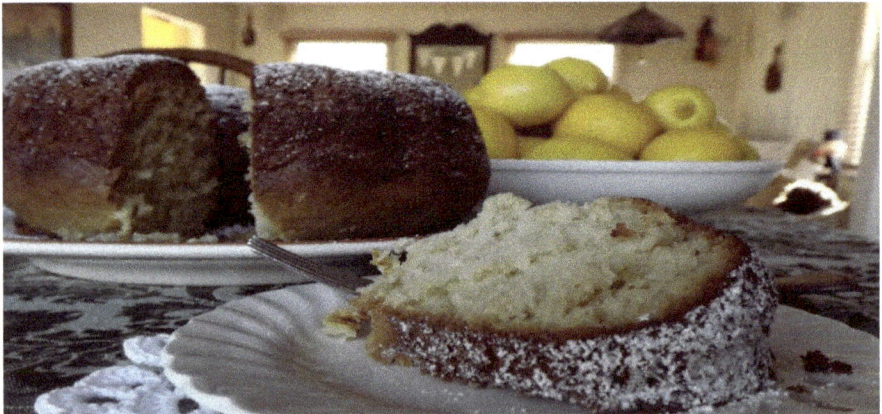

Lemonade Ice Pops

Prep Time:
4 hours and 10 minutes
Cook Time:
0 minutes
Serve: 4

Ingredients:

- 1 cup hot water
- 2 cups cold water
- 2 iced tea and lemonade tea bags

Directions:

1.Put hot water in a container, put in tea bags, cover, and set aside for about ten minutes to steep.

2.Squeeze the tea bags to take off all the water and then discard them. Put in cold water, split into your ice pop maker, freeze for around six hours, before you serve.

Nutrition: ‖ Calories: 38 ‖ Fat: 0 ‖ Fiber: 0 ‖ Carbohydrates: 0 ‖ Protein: 1

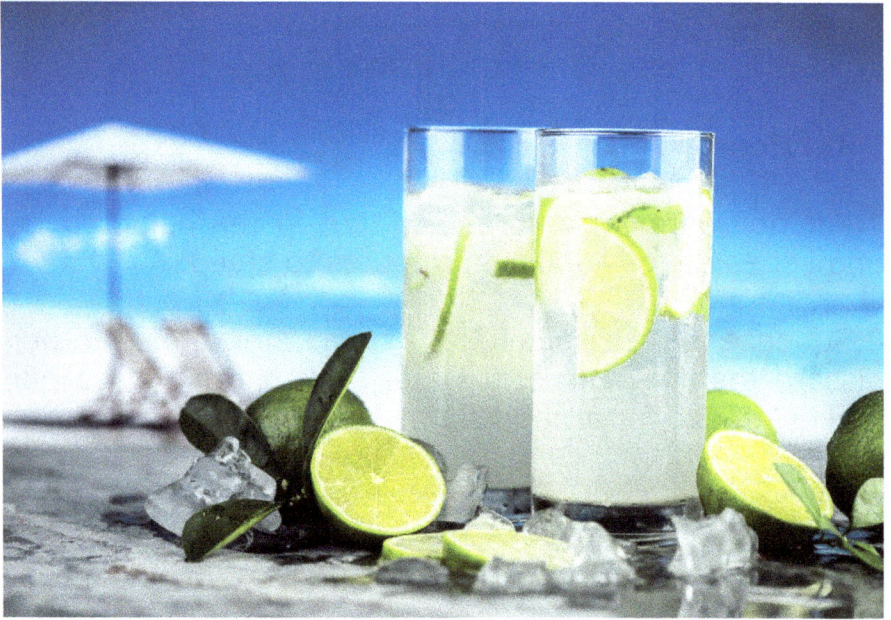

Matcha And Blueberries Pudding

Prep Time:
3 hours
Cook Time:
0 minutes
Serve: 2

Ingredients:

- 1 banana, cut
- 1 cup blueberries
- 1 cup matcha green tea powder
- 2 cups almond milk
- 4 tablespoons chia seeds

Directions:

1.Put chia seeds, milk and matcha powder in a container. Stir, cover, then place in your fridge for around three hours.

2.Split into bowls, top with banana slices and blueberries before you serve.

Nutrition: ‖ Calories: 324 ‖ Fat: 9 ‖ Fiber: 18 ‖ Carbohydrates: 24 ‖ Protein: 8

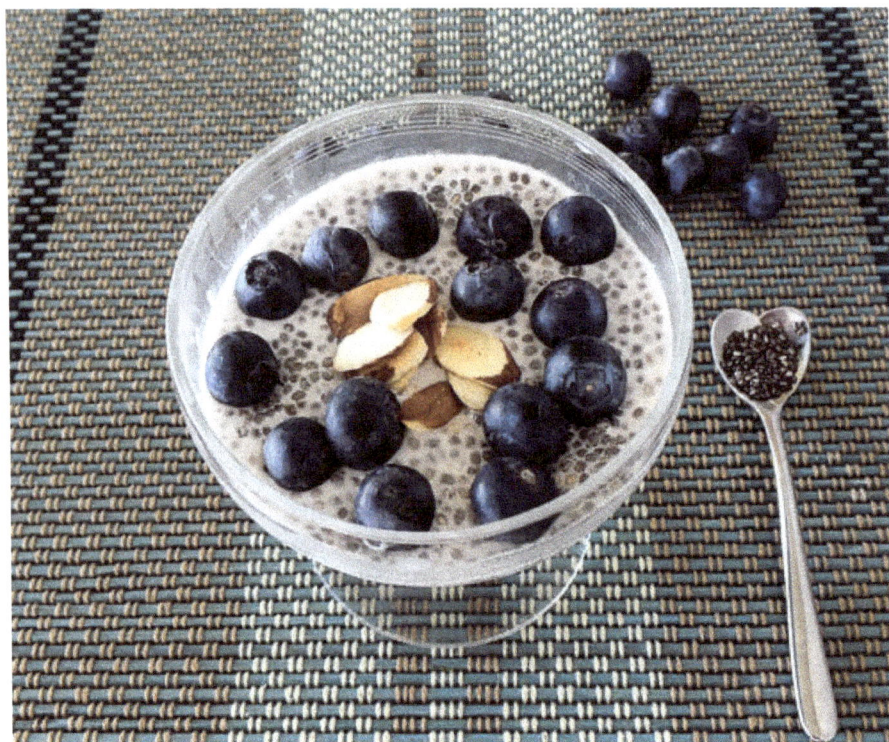

Mediterranean Rolled Baklava With Walnuts

Prep Time:
20 minutes
Cook Time:
40 minutes
Serve: 12

Ingredients:

- 1 cup Cream of wheat or plain breadcrumbs
- 1 Lemon zest
- 1 medium Lemon
- 1/3 cup Milk
- 2 cups Walnuts
- 3 cups Granulated sugar
- 3 cups Water
- 3 sticks Melted Unsalted butter
- 3 tbsp. Sugar
- 8 sheets Thawed phyllo dough Syrup

Directions:

1.Mix 3 cups of sugar, 3 cups of water and lemon slices in a pan and leave to boil

2.Reduce the heat, then allow it to simmer until the sugar completely dissolves. It should take fifteen minutes. You should have a nice smooth syrup now. Now allow to cool for a bit.

3.Cut the walnuts in a blender into bits using short pulses.

4.Pour the walnuts in a container together with the cream of wheat, lemon zest and 4 tablespoons of sugar.

5.Mix in milk and save for later.

6.Now, preheat the oven to 375°F.

7.Spread out the phyllo dough and fit it into a baking pan. Trim off the edges that do not fit with scissors. Cover the rest of the phyllo sheets while you work so they do not dry out.

8.Put a sheet on a clean flat surface and glaze with melted butter. Do this for all the sheets until it's finished.

9.Position the walnut mixture on one side of the sheets and roll them up like you're trying to make a sausage. Do this for all the sheets and walnuts.

10.Position the walnut rolls on an ungreased baking pan and glaze with the leftover butter.

11.Bake for approximately 45 minutes. It's ready when it looks golden.

12.Turn off the oven then pull out the baking pan. Sprinkle syrup over the baklava, ensuring the syrup gets everywhere.

13.Bring back the baking pan into the oven then let sit for five minutes.

14.Remove from the oven and allow to cool for a few hours. Cut the rolls into small amounts before you serve.

Nutrition: ‖ Calories: 488 kcal ‖ Protein: 4.49 g ‖ Fat: 36.89 g ‖ Carbohydrates: 38.21 g

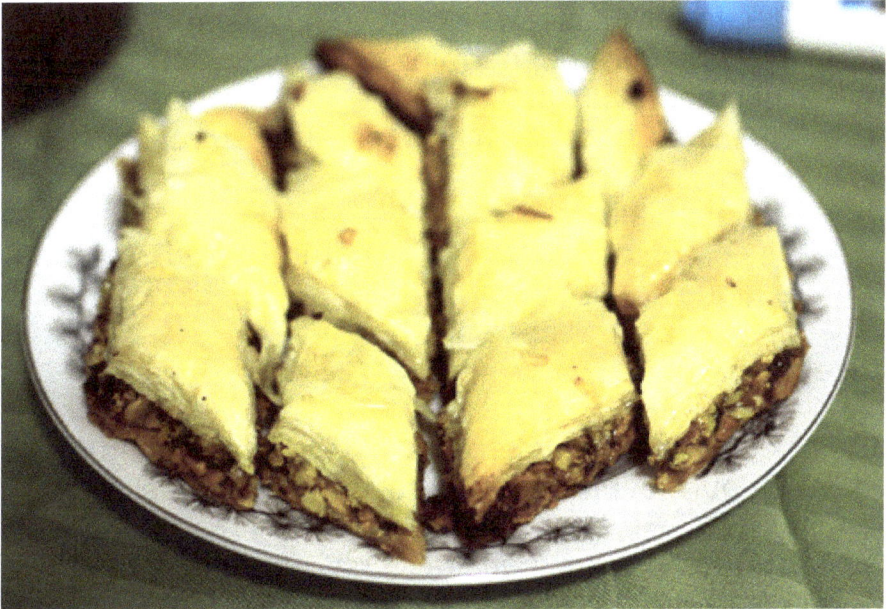

Mint Chocolate Chip Ice-Cream

Prep Time:
5 minutes
Cook Time:
0 minutes
Serve: 2

Ingredients:

- ½ cup Raw cashews or coconut cream, optional.
- 1/8 tsp. Pure peppermint extract
- 2 Frozen overripe bananas
- 3 tbsp. Chocolate chips or sugar-free chocolate chips
- A pinch Salt
- Pinch Spirulina or any natural food coloring, optional.

Directions:

1.Mint or imitation peppermint won't be a substitute for this. Use pure peppermint extract and pour in slowly.

2.Peel and chop the bananas first. Put the slices in a Ziplock bag then freeze.

3.For the ice cream, put all the ingredients in a blender and pulse. You can skip the chocolate chips and just put in them after blending.

4.Serve the moment it's ready or freeze until it's firm enough.

Nutrition: ‖ Calories: 250 kcal ‖ Protein: 6.13 g ‖ Fat: 24.37 g ‖ Carbohydrates: 7.72 g

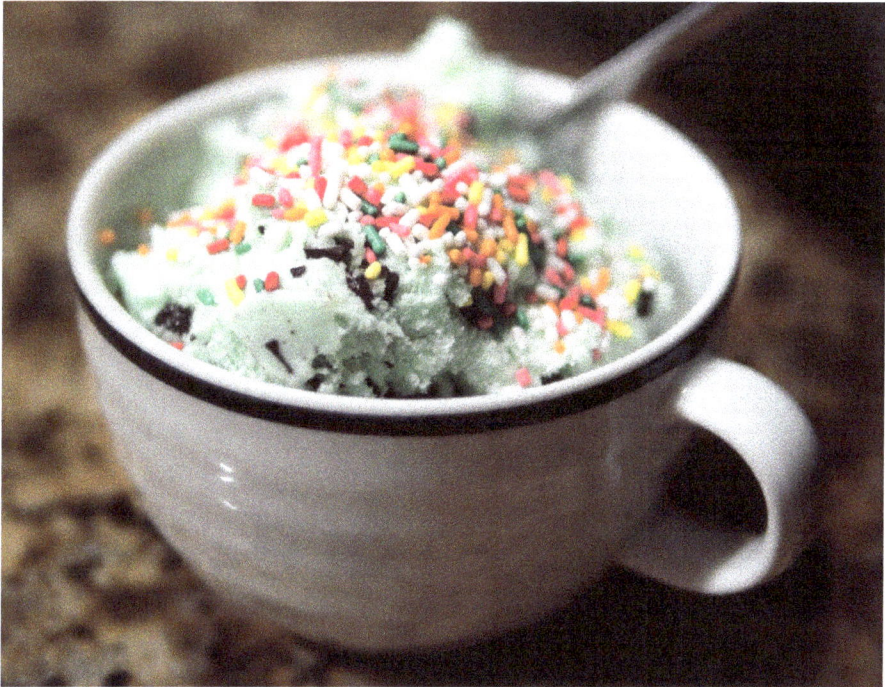

No-Bake Carrot Cake Bites

Prep Time:
15 minutes
Cook Time:
0 minutes
Serve: 6

Ingredients:

- ½ teaspoon of ground ginger
- ¾ cup of shredded coconut
- 1 and a ½ cups of carrots
- 1 cup of pitted Medjool dates
- 1 cup of walnuts
- 1 tablespoon of pure maple syrup
- 1 teaspoon of cinnamon

Directions:

1.Put all together the ingredients into a high-speed blender or food processor, and blend until the mixture comes together, putting in a teaspoon of water at a time if required.

2.Take the carrot mixture and press down into a cupcake tin, and place in your fridge until firm.

3.Pop the carrot cakes out of the muffin tin, and enjoy!

Nutrition: ‖ Total Carbohydrates: 32g ‖ Fiber: 5g ‖ Net Carbohydrates: ‖ Protein: 3g ‖ Total Fat: 12g ‖ Calories: 231

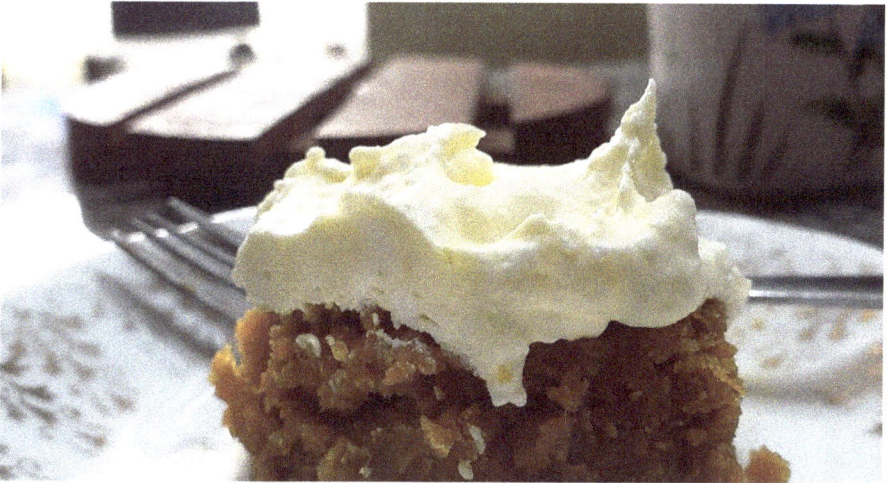

No-Bake Cheesecake

Prep Time:
20 minutes
Cook Time:
0 minutes
Serve: 12

Ingredients:

For Crust:

- 1 cup of dates (pitted and chopped)
- 1 cup of raw almonds
- two to three tablespoons of unsweetened coconut, shredded

For Filling:

- ½ cup of coconut oil, melted
- ¾ cup of fresh lemon juice
- ¾ cup of raw honey
- 1 teaspoon of organic vanilla extract
- 10 drops of liquid stevia
- 2 tablespoons of fresh lemon rind, grated finely
- 3½ cups of cashews, soaked overnight
- A thinly cut lemon Salt

Directions:

1. Put together the dates, almonds, and coconut in a blender and pulse.

2. Move the puree a greased springform pan.

3. Smooth the outer lining of the crust using a spatula.

4.Put cashews and oil in a food processor and pulse.

5.Put in the rest of the ingredients except for lemon slices and pulse until it turns creamy and smooth.

6.Put the combination over the crust uniformly.

7.Smooth the counter of filling using the corner of a spatula.

8.Place in your fridge for one hour.

9.Take it off from the fridge and decorate with lemon slices.

10.Chop it into desired sized slices before you serve.

Nutrition: ‖ Calories: 468 ‖ Fat: 32g ‖ Carbohydrates: 6.6g ‖ Sugar: 44.1g ‖ Protein: 8.4g ‖ Sodium: 23mg

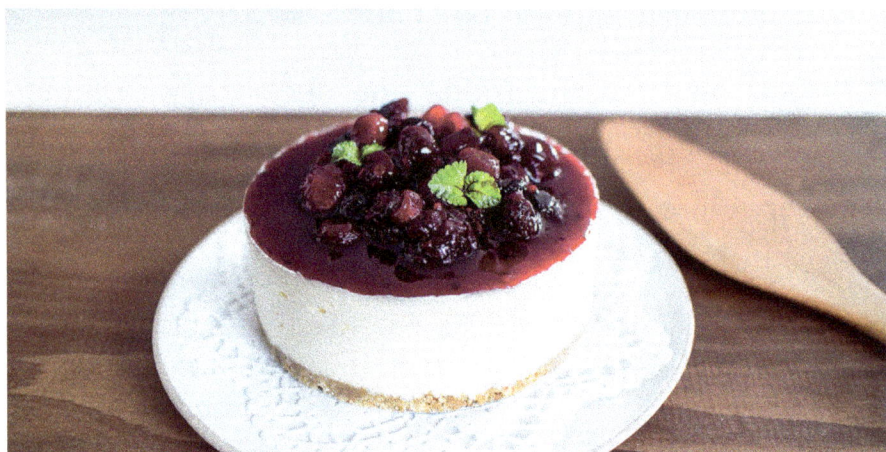

Paleo Raspberry Cream Pie

Prep Time:
20 minutes
Cook Time:
0 minutes
Serve: 12

Ingredients:

For the crust:

- ½ cup Unsweetened shredded coconut
- 1 ½ tbsp. Maple syrup
- 1 cup Roasted or salted cashews
- 1 tsp. Vanilla extract
- Pinch Salt

Raspberry filling:

- ¼ cup & 2 tsp.
- Fresh lemon juice
- ¼ cup Coconut cream from the top solid part of a can of coconut milk that has been placed in the fridge overnight
- ½ cup & 1 tbsp. Maple syrup
- ¾ cup Unrefined coconut oil
- 1 ½ cup Roasted or salted cashews
- 2 tsp. Vanilla extract
- 3 cups Fresh raspberries
- Pinch Salt

Directions:

1.Prepare 12 muffin pans, line them with muffin liners, and set them aside.

2.Make the crust. Set a pan on moderate heat and the coconut and stir until it's completely toasted. Stay by the pan because coconuts tend to burn very easily.

3.Move the toasted coconuts to a container and leave to cool for five minutes or so. Honestly, this toasting step isn't particularly necessary, but I feel it adds amazing flavor to the crust.

4.To make the crust, put all the ingredients in a blender and pulse at the lowest speed until the mix gets all clumpy. Also, do not pulse for too long, or you might end up with a paste.

5.To know if it's ready, put a small amount of the mixture on your fingers and pinch. If it gets clumpy, you're on track, if not, put in a little water and pulse at the lowest speed for further minutes.

6.Scoop the mix into the lined tins using your fingers to pack the mix firmly inside the pan.

7.Place the pans to place in your fridge while you get to make the filling.

8.In a tiny pot set using low heat, mix in all the ingredients until the oil and coconut cream melts completely. Clean the blender using a paper towel and pour in the filling.

9.Pulse at high-speed for like 60 seconds or until it's super smooth. The only clumps we can forgive are the raspberry seeds.

10.Sprinkle a quarter of the filling over the top of each crust. There must be extra filling; you can store and use that in a different dish.

11.Put the coated muffins in your refrigerator to cool. This will take a few hours, like 6 hours, so if you do not have time for that, put it in the freezer.

12.To serve, allow them to defrost for 80 minutes or until obviously creamy.

Nutrition: ‖ Calories: 565 kcal ‖ Protein: 7.74 g ‖ Fat: 43.72 g ‖ Carbohydrates: 42.72 g

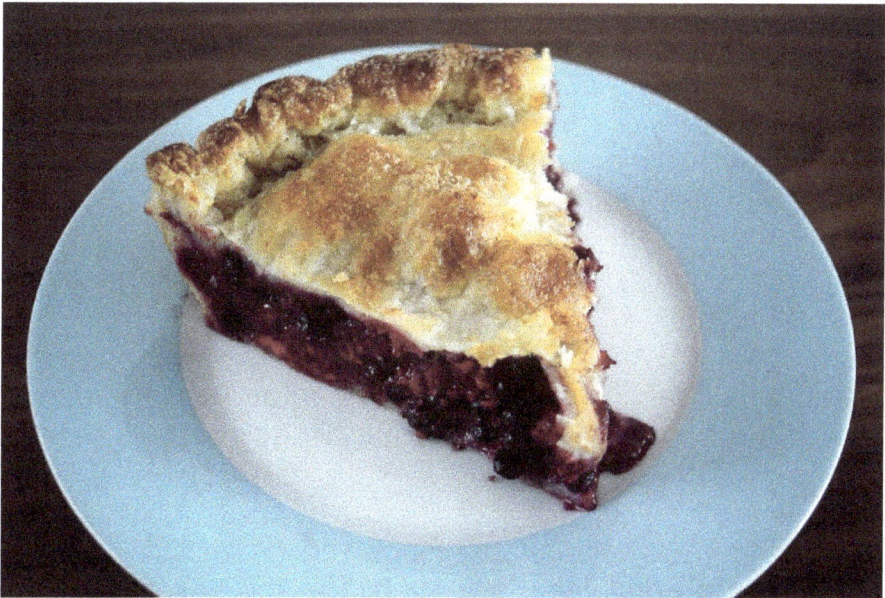

Peanut Butter Balls

Prep Time:
20 minutes
Cook Time:
30 minutes
Serve: 5

Ingredients:

- 1 Tsp. Vanilla Extract
- 2 Tbsp. Peanut Oil.
- 200g Powdered Sugar
- 250g Chocolate
- 250g Creamy Peanut Butter
- 90g Melted Butter

Directions:

1.Mix everything apart from the oil and chocolates to make a batter

2.Place in your fridge the batter for about forty-five minutes.

3.Make small balls with the batter using and put them on a parchment paper. Place in your fridge for one more hour.

4.Melt some dark chocolate. Place the peanut balls into the chocolate and place in your fridge for about twenty minutes.

5.Serve with strawberry.

Nutrition: ‖ Calories: 340 kcal ‖ Carbohydrates: 32 g ‖ Fat: 21 g ‖ Protein: 1.4 g.

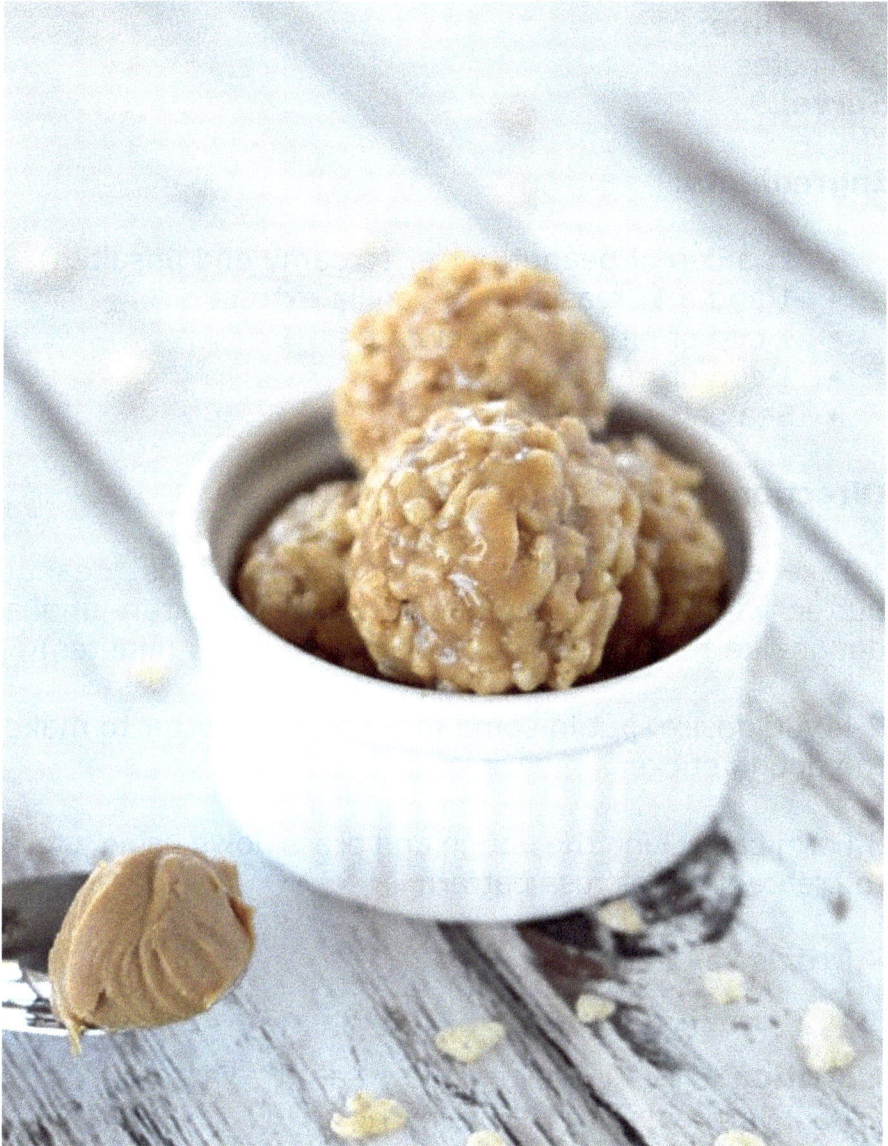

Peanut Butter Cookies

Prep Time:
15 minutes
Cook Time:
0 minutes
Serve: 9

Ingredients:

- ½ a cup of peanut butter (creamy and unsalted)
- 1 and a ¼ teaspoon of vanilla extract
- 1 cup of pitted Medjool dates
- 1 cup of raw almonds
- Sea salt as required

Directions:

1.Take a food processor and put in almonds, peanut butter, vanilla, dates and blend the whole mixture until a dough-like texture comes (should take a few minutes)

2.If you desire, put in some more peanut butter to make the dough sticker.

3.Form balls using the dough and press down using a fork to create a criss-cross pattern

4.Drizzle salt liberally

Nutrition: ‖ Calories: 350 Cal ‖ Fat: 17 g ‖ Carbohydrates: 27 g ‖ Protein: 18 g

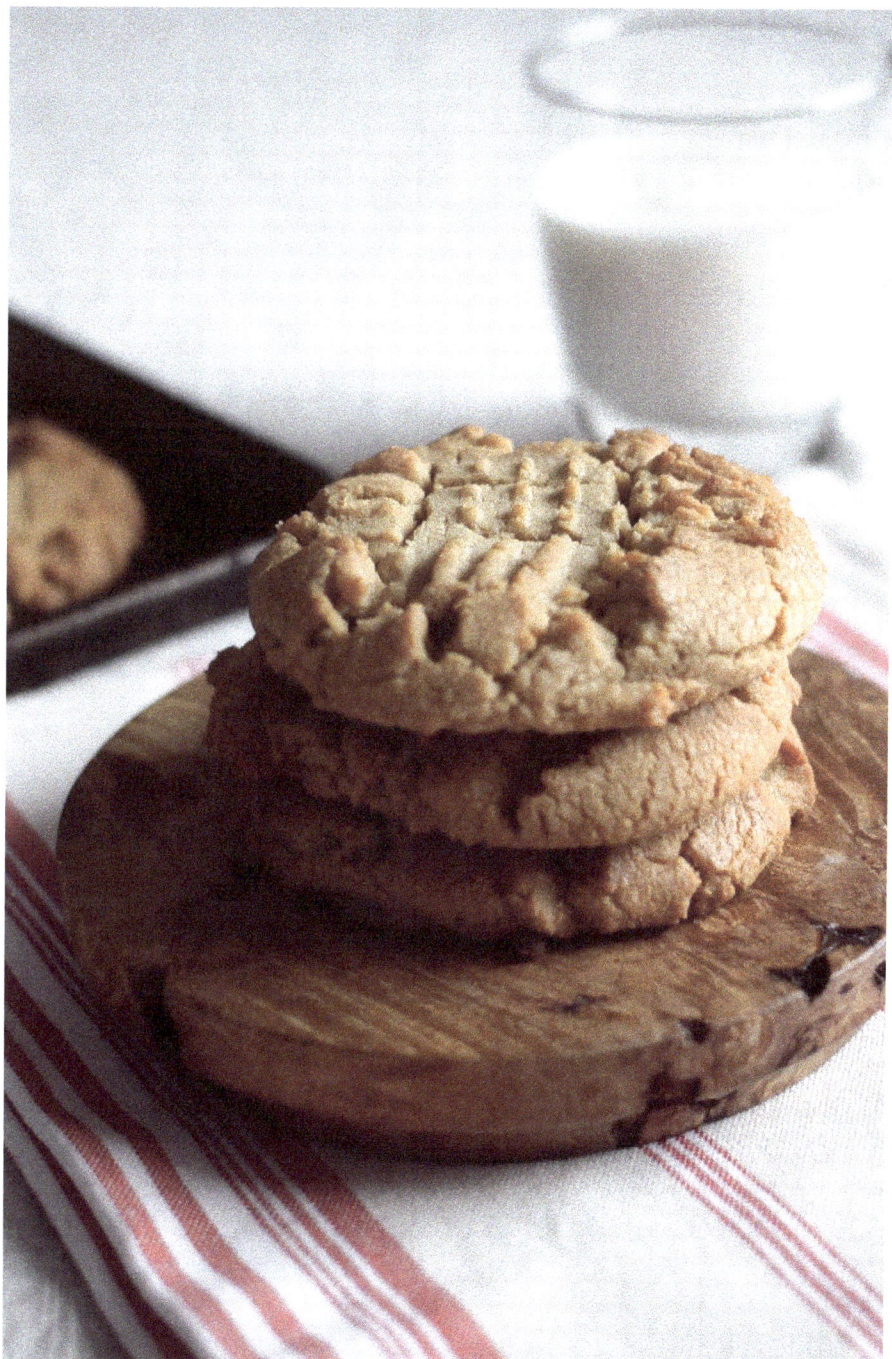

Pineapple Cake

Prep Time:
15 minutes
Cook Time:
50 minutes
Serve: 8

Ingredients:

- ½ tsp. Baking powder
- 1 tbsp. Almond flour
- 1 tsp. Vanilla extract
- 2 slices Fresh pineapples
- 2 Whole medium eggs
- 3 tbsp. Melted coconut oil
- 5 tbsp. Raw honey
- fifteen pcs. Frozen sweet cherries

Directions:

1.Preheat your oven to 350°F.

2.Take away the skin and core of the pineapples. Set aside.

3.Sprinkle 1½ tablespoons of raw honey in a round cake tin.

4.Layer the pineapple rings and sweet cherries on the honey in a decorative fashion.

5.Bring the cake tin in your oven then bake for fifteen minutes.

6.While all that is going on, mix in the almond and baking powder.

7.In a different container, mix the eggs and leftover honey. Sprinkle in coconut oil and stir.

8.Now put in the almond mix to the egg mix and stir meticulously.

9.Take out the cake tin and sprinkle batter over the top of the partly baked pineapple rings and use a spatula to spread it uniformly.

10.Place the cake tin back in your oven and bake for an additional thirty-five minutes.

11.When it's all set, take it out of the oven and leave it to sit for about ten minutes before place it to a plate.

12.Serve with extra cherries if you prefer.

Nutrition: ‖ Calories: 120 kcal ‖ Protein: 2.3 g ‖ Fat: 6.99 g ‖ Carbohydrates: 12.98 g

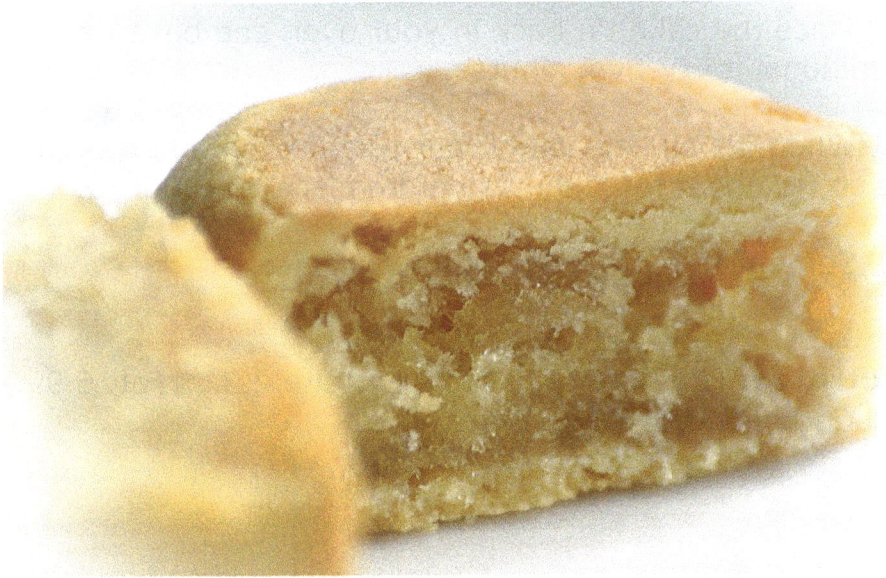

Pineapple Pie

Prep Time:
15 minutes
Cook Time:
50 minutes
Serve: 8

Ingredients:

- ½-tsp baking powder
- 1-cup almond flour
- 1-tsp pure vanilla extract
- 2-pcs eggs
- 2-pcs fresh pineapple, peeled, cored, and cut into rings
- 3-Tbsps liquid coconut oil
- 5-Tbsps raw honey (divided)
- fifteen-pcs sweet cherries, fresh or frozen

Directions:

1.Preheat the oven to 350 °F.

2.Pour 1½-tablespoon of the honey in a round baking tin. Position the cherries and pineapple rings on the bed of honey in a decorative pattern. Put the pan in your oven, then bake for minimum fifteen minutes.

3.Meanwhile, mix in all the rest of the ingredients in a mixing container. Mix thoroughly until forming the mixture into dough. Set aside.

4.Take the pan out from the oven. Push down the batter over the pineapple rings, smoothing it at the top.

5.Return the pan in your oven, and bake further for a little more than half an hour.

Nutrition: ‖ Calories: 213 ‖ Fat: 7.1g ‖ Protein: 15.9g ‖ Sodium: 39.2mg ‖ Total Carbohydrates: 23.7g ‖ Fiber: 2.4g ‖ Net Carbohydrates: 21.3g

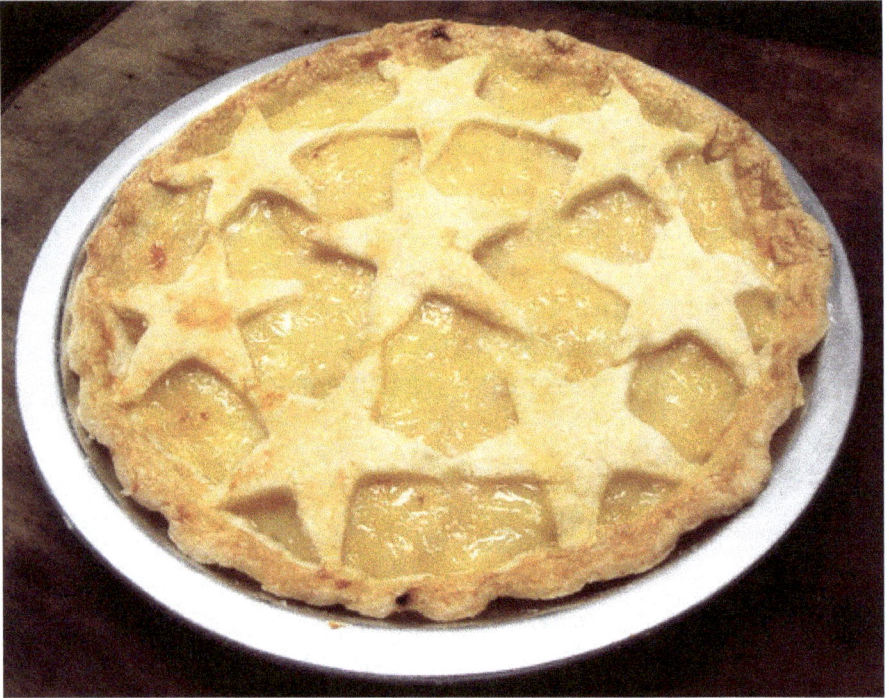

Pistachioed Panna-Cotta Cocoa

Prep Time:
18 minutes
Cook Time:
2 minutes
Serve: 6

Ingredients:

- 12-oz. dark chocolate
- 1-Tbsp coconut oil
- 3-pcs big bananas, cut into thirds Cocoa nibs, chopped
- Salted pistachios, chopped
- Spiced or smoked almonds, chopped

Directions:

1.Coat a baking pan using parchment paper.

2.Melt the dark chocolate with oil in your microwave. Set aside.

3.Pierce a Popsicle stick midway into one end of each banana.

4.Immerse each banana into the melted chocolate. Put dipped bananas into the baking sheet. Drizzle liberally with the cocoa nibs, almonds, and pistachios. Put the sheet in your freezer to harden and set.

Nutrition: ‖ Calories: 454 ‖ Fat: 15.1g ‖ Protein: 22.7g ‖ Sodium: 91mg ‖ Total Carbohydrates: 61.6g ‖ Fiber: 4.9g ‖ Net Carbohydrates: 56.7g

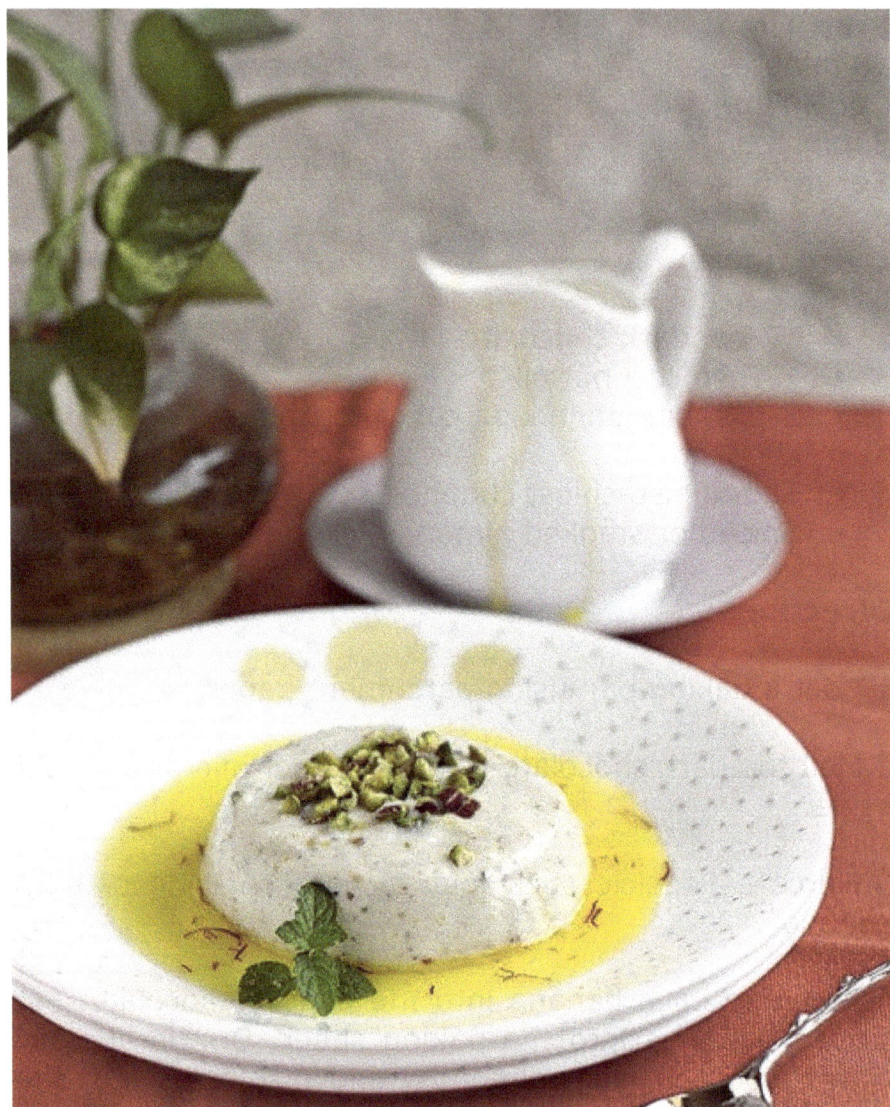

Pumpkin Ice Cream

Prep Time:
15 minutes
Cook Time:
0 minutes
Serve: 6

Ingredients:

- ½ cup of dates (pitted and chopped)
- ½ teaspoon of ground cinnamon
- ½ teaspoon of vanilla flavor
- 1 (fifteen-ounce) can of sugar-free pumpkin puree
- 1 ½ teaspoon of pumpkin pie spice
- 2 (14-ounce) cans of unsweetened coconut milk
- Pinch of salt

Directions:

1.Combine all ingredients in a high-speed blender and pulse.

2.Move the puree to an airtight container and freeze for roughly 1-2 hours.

3.Move the frozen puree to an ice-cream maker and process following the manufacturers.

4.Return the ice-cream to the airtight container and freeze for approximately 1-2 hours before serving.

Nutrition: ‖ Calories: 373 ‖ Fat: 31.9g ‖ Carbohydrates: 24.7g ‖ Sugar: 16.2g ‖ Protein: 4.2g ‖ Sodium: 51mg

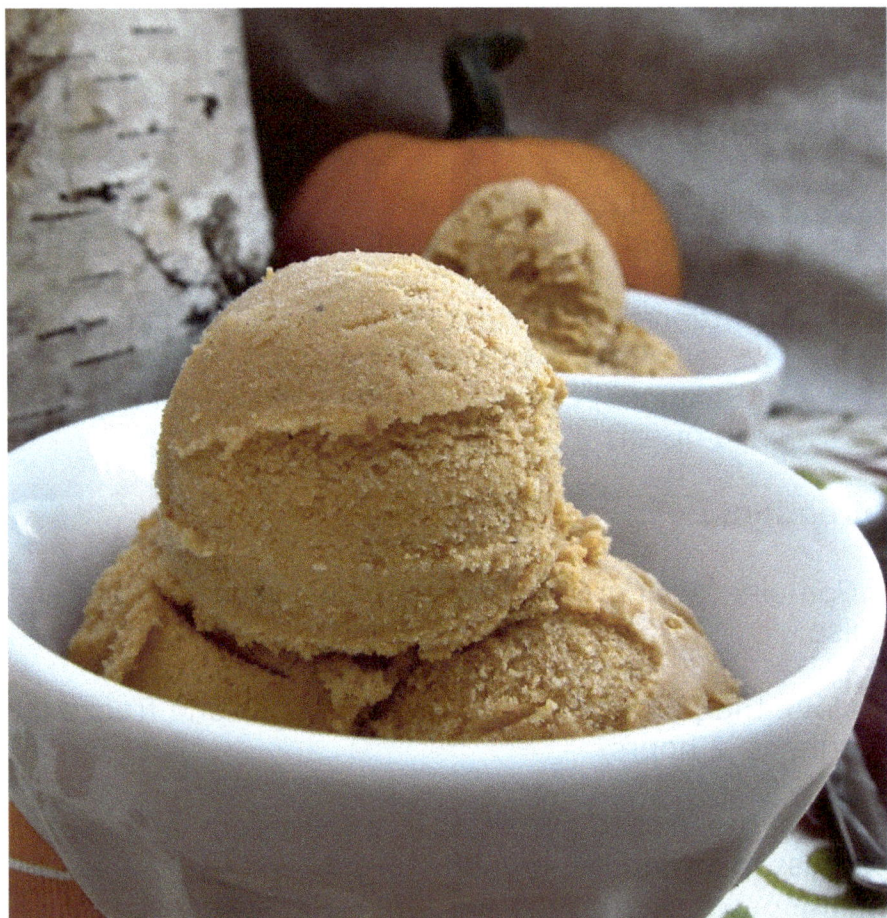

Pure Avocado Pudding

Prep Time:
3 hours
Cook Time:
0 minutes
Serve: 4

Ingredients:

- ¼ teaspoon cinnamon
- ¾ cup cocoa powder
- 1 cup almond milk
- 1 teaspoon vanilla extract
- 2 avocados, peeled and pitted
- 2 tablespoons stevia Walnuts, chopped for serving

Directions:

1.Put in avocados to a blender and pulse well

2.Put in cocoa powder, almond milk, stevia, vanilla bean extract and pulse the mixture well

3.Put into serving bowls then top with walnuts

4.Chill for two to three hours and serve!

Nutrition: ‖ Calories: 221 ‖ Fat: 8g ‖ Carbohydrates: 7g ‖ Protein: 3g

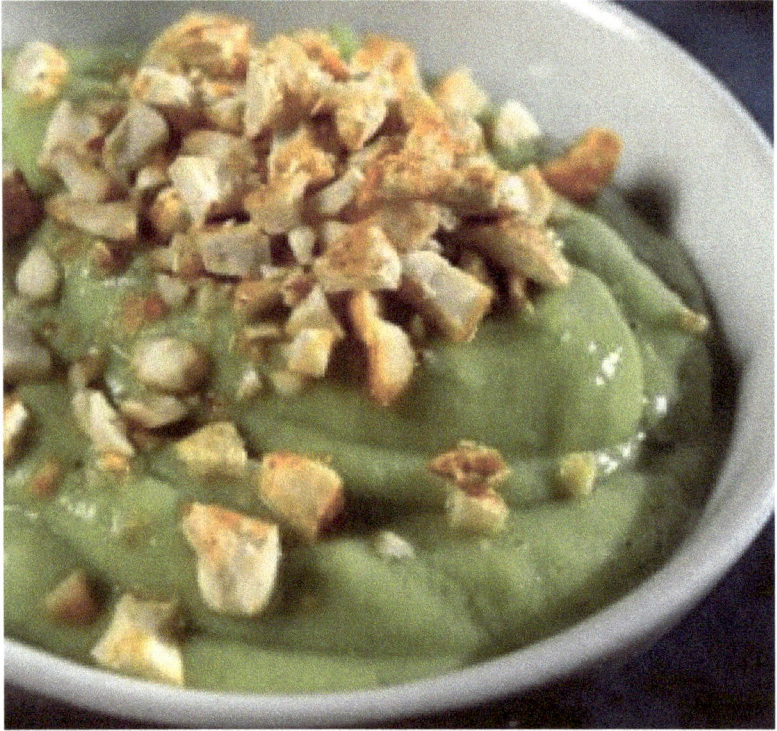

Raspberry Diluted Frozen Sorbet

Prep Time:
10 minutes
Cook Time:
20 minutes
Serve: 4

Ingredients:

- 1 tsp honey
- 14oz / 400g frozen raspberry fl oz /
- 50g almond milk Mint

Directions:

1.Place the almond milk and raspberry in a mixer till it's smooth and leave the consistency in the freezer for about twenty minutes.

2.When serving, place them in ice cream bowls and serve with mint on top

Nutrition: ‖ Calories: 47 ‖ Carbohydrates: 11 g ‖ Protein: 1 g ‖ Fat: 0.4 g ‖ Sugar: 37.2 g ‖ Fiber: 6.0 g ‖ Sodium: 24 mg

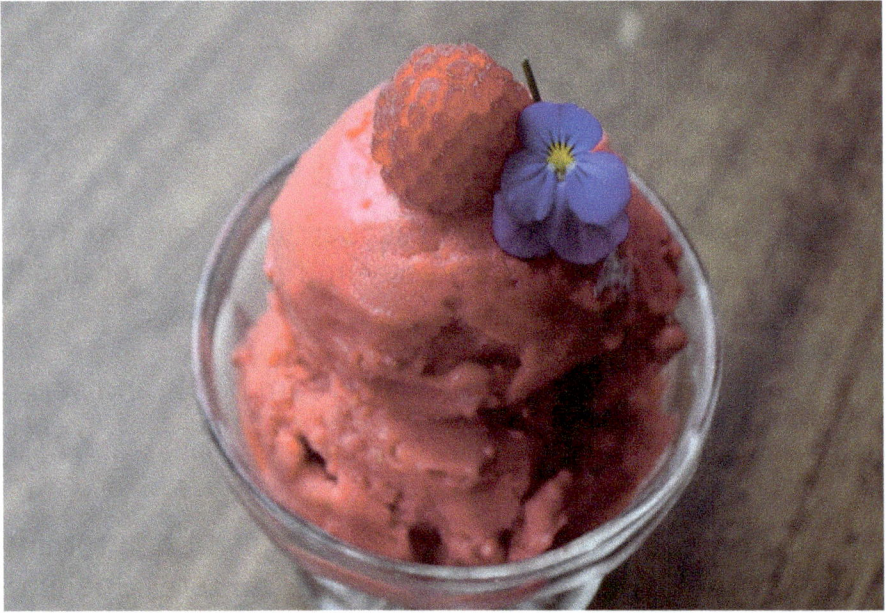

Raspberry Gummies

Prep Time:
5 minutes
Cook Time:
15 minutes
 Serve: 6

Ingredients:

- ¼ cup of grass-fed gelatin
- ¾ cup of cold water
- 1 cup of frozen raspberries
- 3 tablespoons of raw honey

Directions:

1.Put the water and frozen raspberries into a blender, and blend until the desired smoothness is achieved. Put into a big deep cooking pan on moderate heat.

2.Put in the honey and gelatin and whisk together. Reduce the heat, then whisk for another five minutes.

3.Pour into molds or a baking dish, and place in your fridge for minimum 1 hour until firm. If you use a baking dish, chop the gelatin into squares; if not, just pop the gelatin out of the molds.

Nutrition: ‖ Total Carbohydrates: 9g ‖ Fiber: 1g ‖ Net Carbohydrates: ‖ Protein: 0g ‖ Total Fat: 0g ‖ Calories: 37

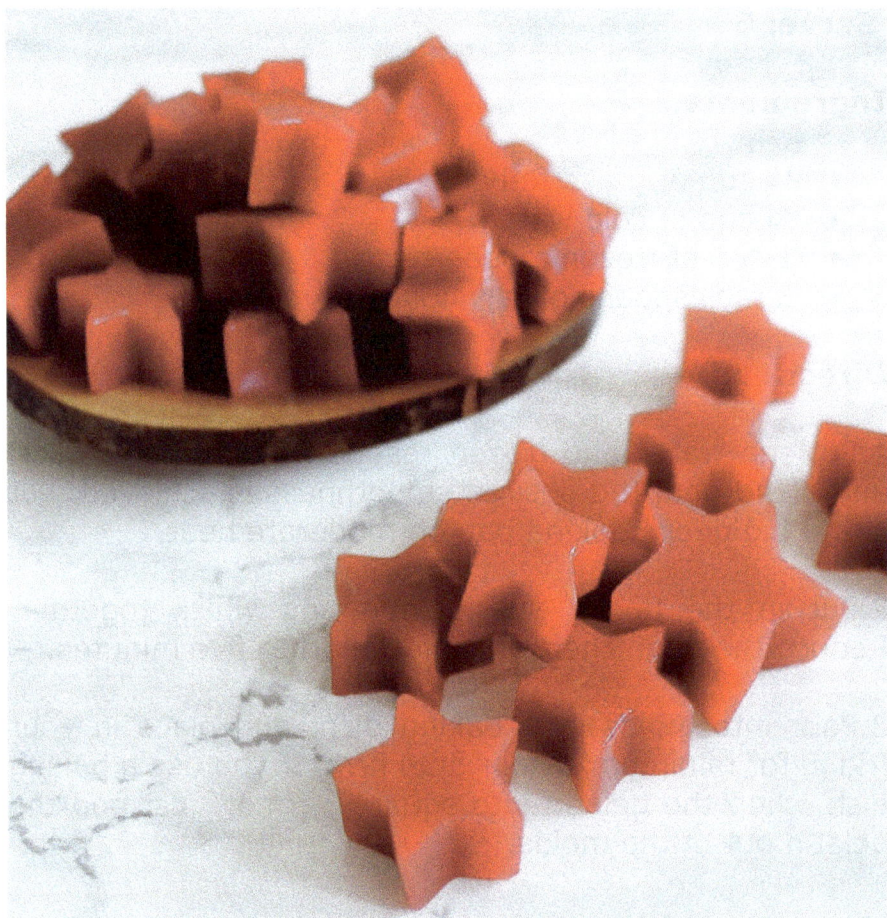

Raw Black Forest Brownies

Prep Time:
2 hours and 10 minutes
Cook Time:
0 minutes
Serve: 6

Ingredients:

- ¼ teaspoon salt
- ½ cup almonds, chopped
- ½ cup dates pitted
- 1 and ½ cups cherries, pitted, dried and chopped
- 1 cup raw cacao powder
- 2 cups walnuts, chopped

Directions:

1.Put all ingredients in a food processor

2.Pulse until small crumbs are formed

3.Push the brownie batter in a pan

4.Freeze for a couple of hours

5.Slice before you serve and enjoy!

Nutrition: ‖ Calories: 294 ‖ Fat: 18g ‖ Carbohydrates: 33g ‖ Protein: 7g

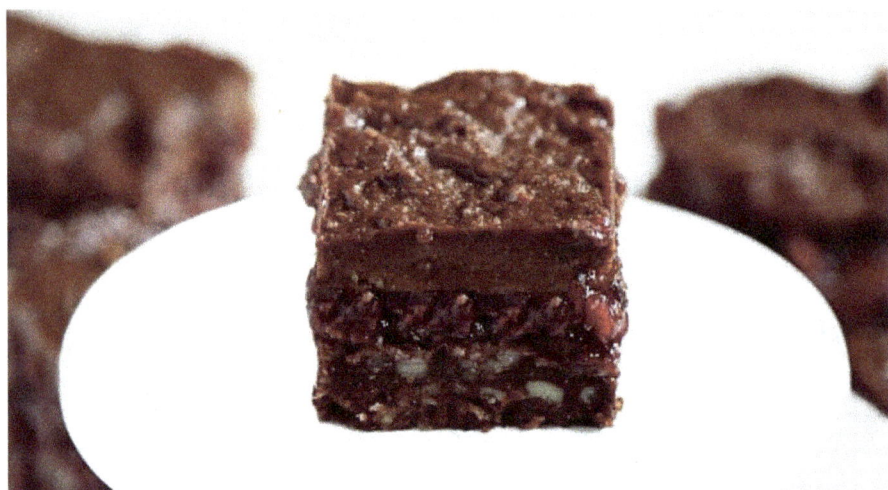

Refreshing Raspberry Jelly

Prep Time:
10 minutes + 1 hours freezing
Cook Time:
30 minutes
Serve: 4

Ingredients:

- ¼ cup of water
- 1 tbsp. of fresh lemon juice
- 2 pound of fresh raspberries

Directions:

1.In a moderate-sized pan, put in raspberries and water on low heat and cook for approximately 8-ten minutes until done completely.

2.Put in lemon juice and cook for approximately 30 minutes, stirring once in a while.

3.Turn off the heat and put the mixture into a sieve.

4.Position a strainer over a container.

5.Through strainer, strain the mixture by pushing using the backside of a spoon.

6.Place the mixture into a blender then pulse till a jelly-like texture is formed.

7.Move into serving glass bowls and place in your fridge for minimum for approximately 1 hour.

Nutrition: ‖ Calories: 119 ‖ Fat: 1.5g ‖ Carbohydrates: 27.2g ‖ Protein: 2.8g ‖ Fiber: 14.8g

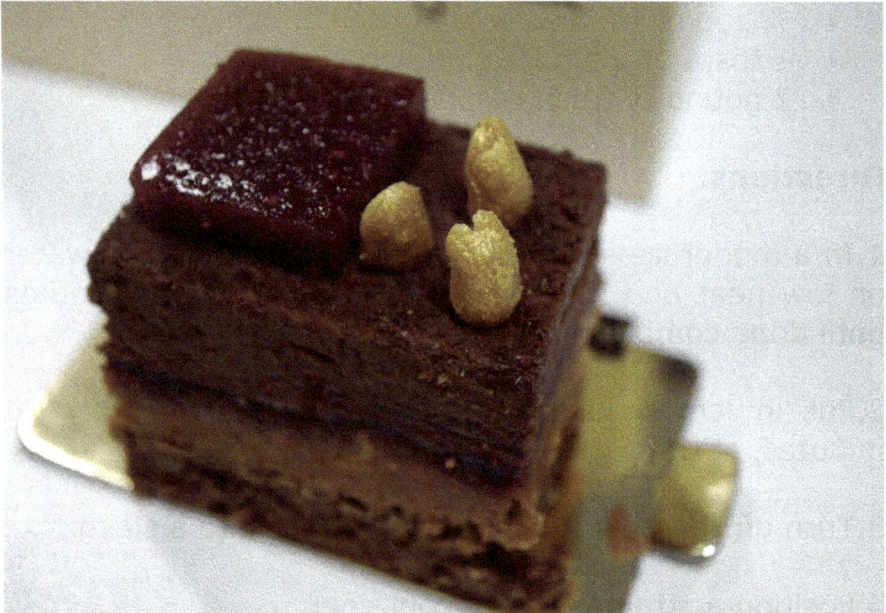

Roasted Bananas

Prep Time:
2 minutes
Cook Time:
7 minutes
Serve: 1

Ingredients:

- 1 banana, cut into diagonal pieces
- Avocado oil cooking spray

Directions:

1.Take parchment paper and line the air fryer basket with it.

2.Preheat the air fryer to 190 degrees C or 375 degrees F.

3.Keep your slices of banana in the basket. Make sure they do not touch

4.Apply avocado oil to mist the slices of banana.

5.Cook for five minutes.

6.Take out the basket. Flip the slices cautiously.

7.Cook for two more minutes. The slices of banana must be caramelized and brown. Remove them from the basket.

Nutrition: Calories 121 ‖ Carbohydrates: 27g ‖ Cholesterol: 0mg ‖ Total Fat: 1g ‖ Protein: 1g ‖ Sugar: 14g ‖ Fiber: 3g ‖ Sodium: 1mg

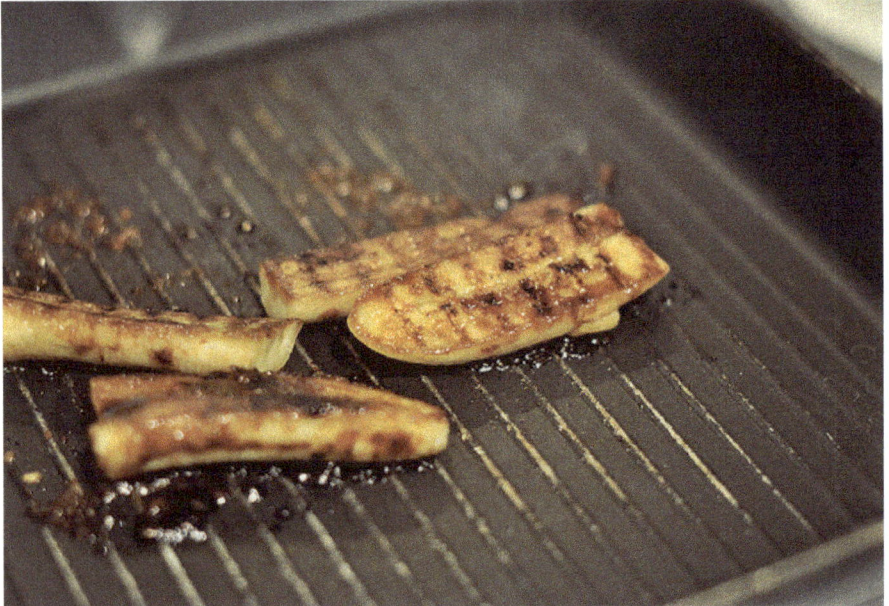

Rum Butter Cookies

Prep Time:
10 minutes + chilling time
Cook Time:
5 minutes
Serve: 12

Ingredients:

- ½ cup coconut butter
- ½ cup confectioners' Swerve
- 1 stick butter
- 1 teaspoon rum extract
- 4 cups almond meal

Directions:

1.Melt the coconut butter and butter. Mix in the Swerve and rum extract.

2.Afterward, put in in the almond meal and mix to blend.

3.Roll the balls and put them on a parchment-lined cookie sheet.

4.Keep in your fridge until ready to serve.

Nutrition: 400 Calories 40g ‖ Fat: 4.9g ‖ Carbs: 5.4g ‖ Protein: 2.9g

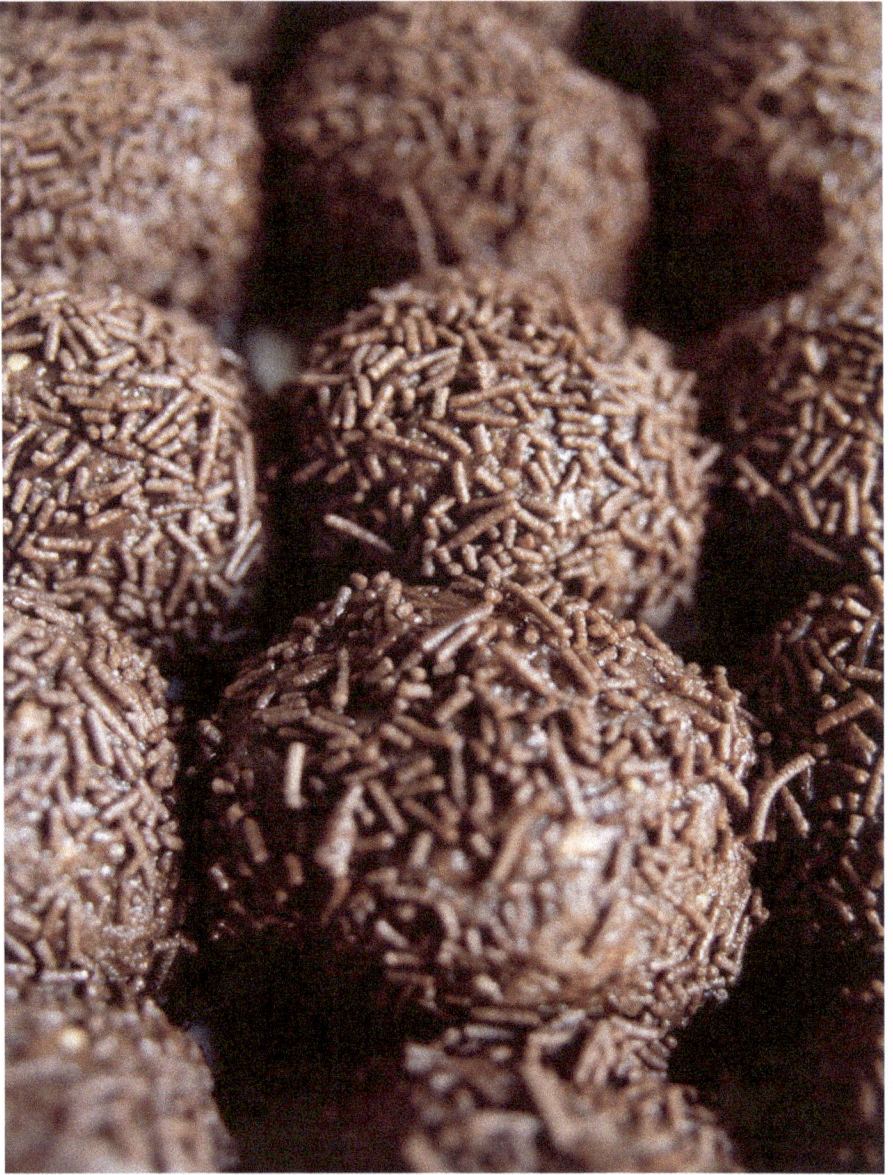

Sherbet Pineapple

Prep Time:
20 minutes
 Cook Time:
0 minutes
Serve: 4

Ingredients:

- 1 can of 8-ounce pineapple chunks
- ¼ teaspoon of ground ginger
- ¼ teaspoon of vanilla extract
- 1 can of 11-ounce orange sections
- 2 cups of pineapple, lemon or lime sherbet
- 1/3 cup of orange marmalade

Directions:

1.Drain the pineapple, ensure you reserve the juice.

2.Take a moderate-sized container and put in pineapple juice, ginger, vanilla and marmalade to the container

3.Put in pineapple chunks, drained mandarin oranges as well

4.Toss thoroughly and coat everything

5.Free them for fifteen minutes and let them chill

6.Ladle the sherbet into 4 chilled stemmed sherbet dishes

7.Top each of them with fruit mixture

Nutrition: ‖ Calories: 267 Cal ‖ Fat: 1 g ‖ Carbohydrates: 65 g ‖ Protein: 2 g

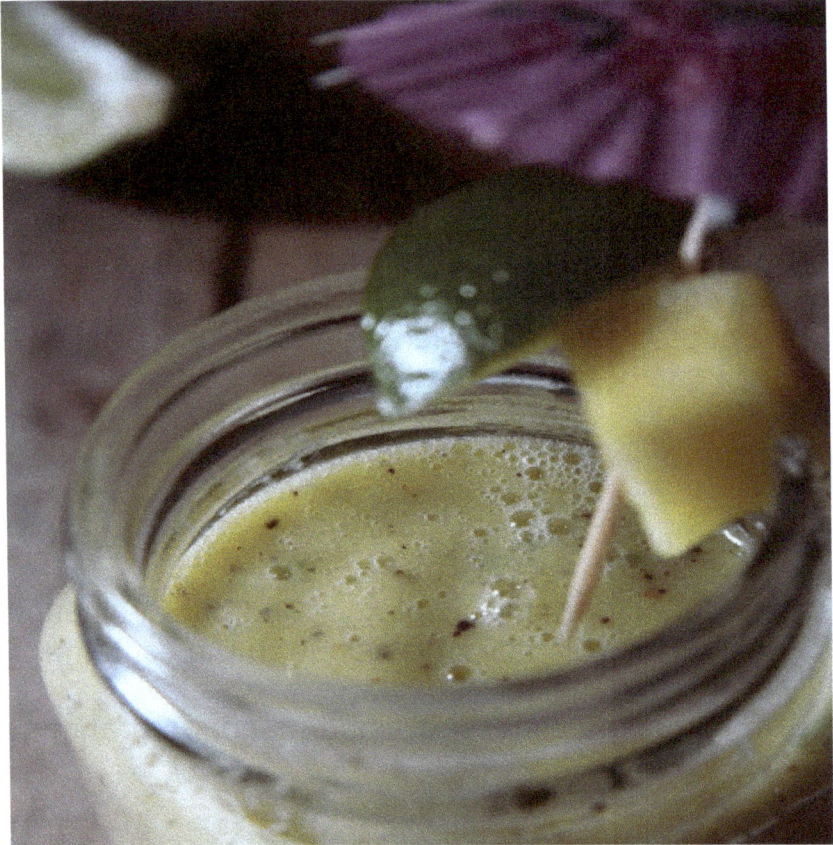

Spiced Tea Pudding

Prep Time:
10 minutes
Cook Time:
10 minutes
Serve: 3

Ingredients:

- ½ cup coconut flakes
- ½ teaspoon cloves
- 1 ½ cups berries
- 1 can coconut milk
- 1 cup almond milk
- 1 tablespoon chia seeds
- 1 tablespoon ground cinnamon
- 1 tablespoon raw honey
- 1 teaspoon allspice
- 1 teaspoon cardamom
- 1 teaspoon green tea powder
- 1 teaspoon nutmeg
- 2 tablespoons pumpkin seeds
- 2 teaspoons ground ginger

Directions:

1.In your blender, puree tea powder with coconut milk, almond milk, cinnamon, coconut flakes, nutmeg, allspice, cloves, honey, cardamom, and ginger split into bowls.

2.Heat a pan on moderate heat, put in berries until bubbling, then move to your blender and pulse well. Split the berries into the bowls with the coconut milk mix, top with chia seeds and pumpkin seeds before you serve.

Nutrition: ‖ Calories: 150 ‖ Fat: 6 ‖ Fiber: 5 ‖ Carbohydrates: 14 ‖ Protein: 8

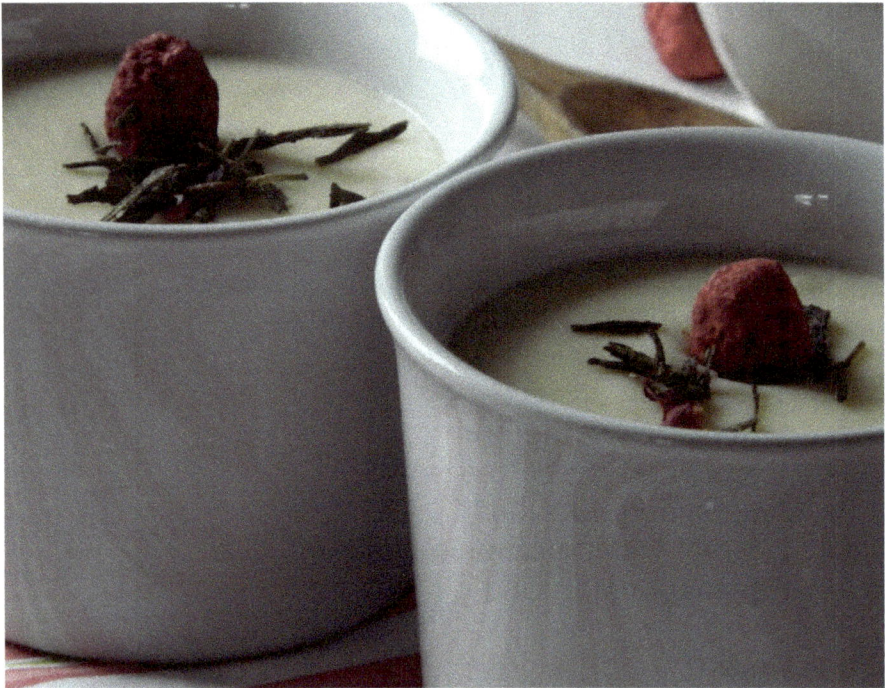

Spicy Popper Mug Cake

Prep Time:
5 minutes
Cook Time:
5 minutes
Serve: 2

Ingredients:

- ¼ teaspoon sunflower seeds
- ½ a jalapeno pepper
- ½ teaspoon baking powder
- 1 bacon, cooked and cut
- 1 big egg
- 1 tablespoon almond butter
- 1 tablespoon cashew cheese
- 1 tablespoon flaxseed meal
- 2 tablespoons almond flour

Directions:

1.Take a frying pan then place it on moderate heat

2.Put cut bacon and cook until they have a crunchy texture

3.Take a microwave proof container and mix all of the listed ingredients (including cooked bacon), clean the sides

4.Microwave for 75 seconds making to put your microwave to high power

5.Take out the cup and slam it against a surface to take the cake out

6.Decorate using a bit of jalapeno and serve!

Nutrition: ‖ Calories: 429 ‖ Fat: 38g ‖ Carbohydrates: 6g ‖ Protein: 16g

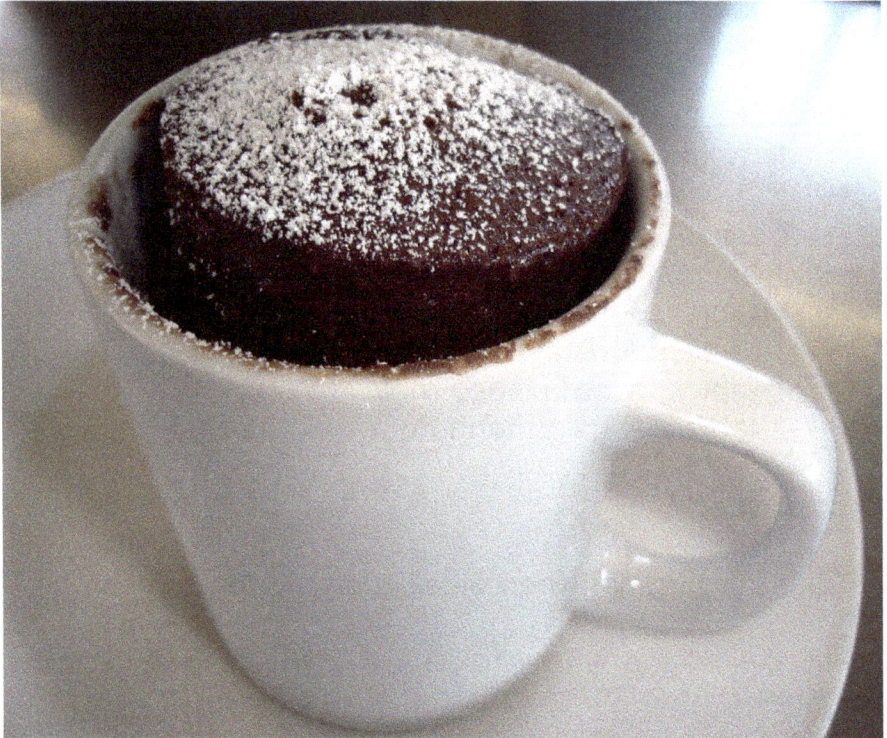

Strawberry Granita

Prep Time:
10 minutes
Cook Time:
10 minutes
Serve: 8

Ingredients:

- ¼ teaspoon balsamic vinegar
- ½ teaspoon lemon juice
- 1 cup of water
- 2 lb. strawberries, halved & hulled
- Agave to taste
- Just a small pinch of salt

Directions:

1.Wash the strawberries in water.

2.Keep in a blender. Put in water, agave, balsamic vinegar, salt, and lemon juice.

3.Pulse multiple times so that the mixture moves. Blend until smooth.

4.Pour into a baking dish. The puree must be 3/8 inch deep only.

5.Place in your fridge the dish uncovered till the edges start to freeze. The center must be slushy.

6.Stir crystals from the edges lightly into the center. Stir thoroughly to mix.

7.Chill till the granite is nearly fully frozen.

8.Scrape loose the crystals like before and mix.

9.Place in your fridge once more. Using a fork, stir 3-4 times till the granite has become light.

Nutrition: Calories 72 || Carbohydrates: 17g || Fat: 0g || Sugar: 14g || Fiber: 2g || Protein: 1g

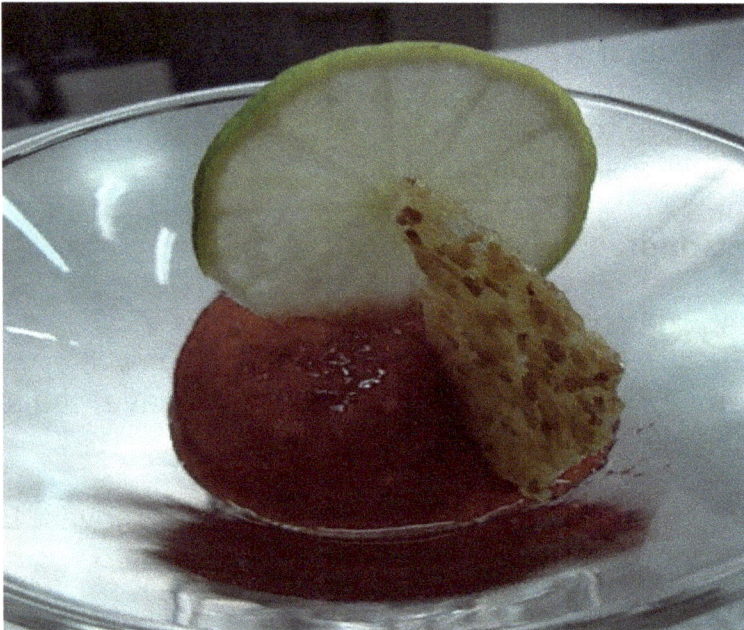